Third Edition

Nursing Professional Development

Review Manual

CONTINUING EDUCATION SOURCE
NURSING CERTIFICATION REVIEW MANUAL
CLINICAL PRACTICE RESOURCE

Ellen Gorbunoff, MSN, RN-BC, and
Patricia Kummeth, MSN, RN-BC

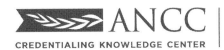

ANCC

CREDENTIALING KNOWLEDGE CENTER | Conferences. Consultation. Education.

Library of Congress Cataloging-in-Publication Data

Gorbunoff, Ellen, author.

Nursing professional development review manual / by Ellen Gorbunoff and Patricia Kummeth.—3rd edition.

    p. ; cm.

Preceded by Nursing professional development : review and resource manual / Diane D. DePew and Patricia Kummeth. 2nd ed. 2011.

Includes bibliographical references and index.

ISBN 978-1-935213-57-4

I. Kummeth, Patricia, author. II. DePew, Diane. Nursing professional development. Preceded by (work): III. American Nurses Credentialing Center, publisher. IV. Title.

[DNLM: 1. Education, Nursing, Continuing--Outlines. 2. Nursing Staff--education—Outlines. 3. Staff Development—methods—Outlines. 4. Teaching—methods—Outlines. WY 18.2]

RT76

610.73071'5--dc23

                    2014020066

The mission of the American Nurses Credentialing Center (ANCC), a subsidiary of the American Nurses Association (ANA), is to promote excellence in nursing and health care globally through credentialing programs. ANCC's internationally renowned credentialing programs certify and recognize individual nurses in specialty practice areas. ANCC recognizes healthcare organizations that promote nursing excellence and quality patient outcomes while providing safe, positive work environments. In addition, ANCC accredits healthcare organizations that provide and approve continuing nursing education. The ANCC Credentialing Knowledge Center™ offers educational materials to support nurses and organizations as they work toward their credentials.

ISBN 13: 978-1-935213-57-4

NURSING PROFESSIONAL DEVELOPMENT REVIEW MANUAL, 3RD EDITION

JULY 2014

Please direct your comments and/or queries to: revmanuals@ana.org

The healthcare services delivery system is a volatile marketplace demanding superior knowledge, clinical skills, and competencies from all registered nurses. Nursing autonomy of practice and nurse career marketability and mobility in the new century hinge on affirming the profession's formative philosophy, which places a priority on a lifelong commitment to the principles of education and professional development. The knowledge base of nursing theory and practice is expanding, and while care has been taken to ensure the accuracy and timeliness of the information presented in the **Nursing Professional Development Review Manual, 3rd Edition,** clinicians are advised to always verify the most current national guidelines and recommendations and to practice in accordance with professional standards of care used with regard to the unique circumstances that apply in each practice situation. In addition, the editors wish to note that provision of information in this text does not imply an endorsement of any particular products, procedures or services.

Therefore, the authors, editors, American Nurses Association (ANA), American Nurses Association's Publishing (ANP), American Nurses Credentialing Center (ANCC), and the Credentialing Knowledge Center cannot accept responsibility for errors or omissions, or for any consequences or liability, injury, and/or damages to persons or property from application of the information in this manual and make no warranty, express or implied, with respect to the contents of the **Nursing Professional Development Review Manual, 3rd Edition**. Completion of this manual does not guarantee that the reader will pass the certification exam. The practice examination questions are not a requirement to take a certification examination. The practice examination questions cannot be used as an indicator of results on the actual certification.

PUBLISHED BY
American Nurses Credentialing Center
Credentialing Knowledge Center
8515 Georgia Avenue, Suite 400
Silver Spring, MD 20910-3402
www.nursecredentialing.org

INTRODUCTION TO THE CONTINUING EDUCATION (CE) CONTACT HOUR APPLICATION PROCESS FOR *NURSING PROFESSIONAL DEVELOPMENT REVIEW MANUAL, 3RD EDITION*

The Credentialing Knowledge Center offers the continuing education contact hours for this manual online at www.NursingWorld.org, the American Nurses Association's website. This process involves answering approximately 25–30 questions that test knowledge of the information contained within this manual. The continuing education contact hours can be completed at any time and a certificate can be printed from the website immediately upon successful completion of the test.

After studying the manual and given an online multiple-choice test, the exam candidate will be able to:

1. Pass the posttest with at least 75% of the answers correct.

2. Select responses to test questions based on key principles, standards of practice, and theoretical basis of nursing practice.

3. Choose accepted therapeutic interventions in answering questions related to quality nursing practice.

4. Utilize direct and indirect professional role responsibilities and applications regarding nursing practice in answering test questions.

Upon completion of this manual and the online CE test, a nurse can receive a total of 21.95 continuing education contact hours at a price of $30. (ANA members receive a discount on CEs.) **The entire process—online test and evaluation form—must be completed by June 30, 2017 in order to receive credi**t. To begin the process, please email revmanuals@ana.org. Your patience with this process is greatly appreciated.

Inquiries or Comments
If you have any questions about the CE contact hours, please email revmanuals@ana.org. You may also mail any comments to Editorial Project Manager at the address listed below.

Duplicate CE Certificates
Once you have successfully passed the CE test, you may go back and re-print your certificate as often as you wish.

Conflicts of Interest

A conflict of interest occurs when an individual has an opportunity to affect educational content about healthcare products or services of a commercial company with which she/he has a financial relationship.

The planners and presenters of this CNE activity have disclosed no relevant financial relationships with any commercial companies pertaining to this activity.

Credentialing Knowledge Center
American Nurses Credentialing Center
Attn: Editorial Project Manager
8515 Georgia Avenue, Suite 400
Silver Spring, MD 20910-3492
Fax: (301) 628-5342

A maximum of 21.95 contact hours may be earned by learners who successfully complete this continuing nursing education activity.

The American Nurses Association Center for Continuing Education and Professional Development is accredited as a provider of continuing nursing education by the American Nurses Credentialing Center's Commission on Accreditation.

ANCC Provider Number 0023.

ANA is approved by the California Board of Registered Nursing, Provider Number CEP6178.

The ANA Center for Continuing Education and Professional Development includes ANCC's Credentialing Knowledge Center.

CONTENTS

CHAPTER 1

TAKING THE CERTIFICATION EXAMINATION

When you sign up to take a national certification exam, you will be instructed to go online and review the testing and review handbook (http://www.nursecredentialing.org/CertificationHandbook.aspx). Review it carefully and be sure to bookmark the site so you can refer to it frequently. It contains information on test content and sample questions. This is critical information; it will give you insight into the nature of the test. The agency will send you information about the test site; keep this in a safe place until needed.

GENERAL SUGGESTIONS FOR PREPARING FOR THE EXAM

Step One: Control Your Anxiety

Everyone experiences anxiety when faced with taking the certification exam.

- ▶ Remember, your program was designed to prepare you to take this exam.

- ▶ Your instructors took a similar exam, and have probably talked to students who took exams more recently, so they know how to help you prepare.

- ▶ Taking a review course or setting up your own study plan will help you feel more confident about taking the exam.

Step Two: Do Not Listen to Gossip About the Exam

A large volume of information exists about the tests based on reports from people who have taken the exams in the past. Because information from the testing facilities is limited, it is hard to ignore this gossip.

▶ Remember that gossip about the exam that you hear from others is not verifiable.

▶ Because this gossip is based on the imperfect memory of people in a stressful situation, it may not be very accurate.

▶ People tend to remember those items testing content with which they are less comfortable; for instance, those with a limited background in women's health may say that the exam was "all women's health." In fact, the exam blueprint ensures that the exam covers multiple content areas without overemphasizing any one.

Step Three: Set Reasonable Expectations for Yourself

▶ Do not expect to know everything.

▶ Do not try to know everything in great detail.

▶ You do not need a perfect score to pass the exam.

▶ The exam is designed for a beginner level—it is testing readiness for *entry-level* practice.

▶ Learn the general rules, not the exceptions.

▶ The most likely diagnoses will be on the exam, not questions on rare diseases or atypical cases.

▶ Think about the most likely presentation and most common therapy.

Step Four: Prepare Mentally and Physically

▶ While you are getting ready to take the exam, take good physical care of yourself.

▶ Get plenty of sleep and exercise, and eat well while preparing for the exam.

▶ These things are especially important while you are studying and immediately before you take the exam.

Step Five: Access Current Knowledge

General Content

You will be given a list of general topics that will be on the exam when you register to take the exam. In addition, examine the table of contents of this book and the test content outline, available at www.nursecredentialing.org.

▶ What content do you need to know?

▶ How well do you know these subjects?

Take a Review Course

▶ Taking a review course is an excellent way to assess your knowledge of the content that will be included in the exam.

▶ If you plan to take a review course, take it well before the exam so you will have plenty of time to master any areas of weakness the course uncovers.

▶ If you are prepared for the exam, you will not hear anything new in the course. You will be familiar with everything that is taught.

▶ If some topics in the review course are new to you, concentrate on these in your studies.

▶ People have a tendency to study what they know; it is rewarding to study something and feel a mastery of it! Unfortunately, this will not help you master unfamiliar content. Be sure to use a review course to identify your areas of strength and weakness, then concentrate on the weaknesses.

Depth of Knowledge

How much do you need to know about a subject?

▶ You cannot know everything about a topic.

▶ Study the information sent to you from the testing agency, what you were taught in school, what is covered in this text, and the general guidelines given in this chapter.

▶ Look at practice tests designed for the exam. Practice tests for other exams will not be helpful.

▶ Consult your class notes or clinical diagnosis and management textbook for the major points about a disease. Additional reference books can be found online at www.nursecredentialing.org.

Step Six: Institute a Systematic Study Plan

Develop Your Study Plan

▶ Write up a formal plan of study.

- » Include topics for study, timetable, resources, and methods of study that work for you.

- » Decide whether you want to organize a study group or work alone.

- » Schedule regular times to study.

- » Avoid cramming; it is counterproductive. Try to schedule your study periods in 1-hour increments.

▶ Identify resources to use for studying. To prepare for the examination, you should have the following materials on your shelf:

- » This review book.

- » Your class notes.

- » Other important sources, including: information from the testing facility, a clinical diagnosis textbook, favorite journal articles, notes from a review course, and practice tests.

- » Consult the bibliography on the test blueprint. When studying less familiar material, it is helpful to study using the same references that the testing center uses.

▶ You will need to know facts and be able to interpret and analyze this information utilizing critical thinking.

Personalize Your Study Plan

▶ How do you learn best?

- » If you learn best by listening or talking, attend a review course or discuss topics with a colleague.

▶ Read everything the test facility sends you as soon as you receive it and several times during your preparation period. It will give you valuable information to help guide your study.

▶ Have a specific place with good lighting set aside for studying. Find a quiet place with no distractions. Assemble your study materials.

Implement Your Study Plan

You must have basic content knowledge. In addition, you must be able to use this information to think critically and make decisions based on facts.

- ▶ Refer to your study plan regularly.

- ▶ Stick to your schedule.

- ▶ Take breaks when you get tired.

- ▶ If you start procrastinating, get help from a friend or reorganize your study plan.

- ▶ It is not necessary to follow your plan rigidly. Adjust as you learn where you need to spend more time.

- ▶ Memorize the basics of the content areas you will be required to know.

Focus on General Material

- ▶ Most of what you need to know is basic material that does not require constant updating.

- ▶ You do not need to worry about the latest information being published as you are studying for the exam. Remember, it can take 6 to 12 months for new information to be incorporated into test questions.

Pace Your Studying

- ▶ Stop studying for the examination when you are starting to feel overwhelmed and look at what is bothering you. Then make changes.

- ▶ Break overwhelming tasks into smaller tasks that you know you can do.

- ▶ Stop and take breaks while studying.

Work With Others

- ▶ Talk with classmates about your preparation for the exam.

- ▶ Keep in touch with classmates, and help each other stick to your study plans.

- ▶ If your classmates become anxious, do not let their anxiety affect you. Walk away if you need to.

- ▶ Do not believe bad stories you hear about other people's experiences with previous exams.

- ▶ Remember, you know as much as anyone about what will be on the next exam!

Consider a Study Group

▶ Study groups can provide practice in analyzing cases, interpreting questions, and critical thinking.

    ▹ You can discuss a topic and take turns presenting cases for the group to analyze.

    ▹ Study groups also can provide moral support and help you continue studying.

Step Seven: Strategies Immediately Before the Exam

Final Preparation Suggestions

▶ Use practice exams when studying to get accustomed to the exam format and time restrictions.

    ▹ Many books that are labeled as review books are simply a collection of examination questions.

    ▹ If you have test anxiety, such practice tests may help alleviate the anxiety.

    ▹ Practice tests can help you learn to judge the time it should take you to complete the exam.

    ▹ Practice tests are useful for gaining experience in analyzing questions.

    ▹ Books of questions may not uncover the gaps in your knowledge that a more systematic content review text will reveal.

    ▹ If you feel that you don't know enough about a topic, refer to a text to learn more. After you feel that you have learned the topic, practice questions are a wonderful tool to help improve your test-taking skill.

▶ Know your test-taking style.

    ▹ Do you rush through the exam without reading the questions thoroughly?

    ▹ Do you get stuck and dwell on a question for a long time?

    ▹ You should spend about 45 to 60 seconds per question and finish with time to review the questions you were not sure about.

    ▹ Be sure to read the question completely, including all four answer choices. Choice "a" may be good, but "d" may be best.

The Night Before the Exam

▶ Be prepared to get to the exam on time.

    ▹ Know the test site location and how long it takes to get there.

    ▹ Take a "dry run" beforehand to make sure you know how to get to the testing site, if necessary.

- Get a good night's sleep.

- Eat sensibly.

- Avoid alcohol the night before.

- Assemble the required material—two forms of identification, pencil, and watch. Both IDs must match the name on the application, and one photo ID is preferred.

  - Know the exam room rules.

  - You will be required to put papers, backpacks, etc., in a corner of the room or in a locker.

  - No water or food will be allowed.

  - You will be allowed to walk to a water fountain and go to the bathroom one at a time.

THE DAY OF THE EXAM

- Get there early. You must arrive to the test center at least 15 minutes before your scheduled appointment time. If you are late, you may not be admitted.

- Think positively. You have studied hard and are well-prepared.

- Remember your anxiety reduction strategies.

Specific Tips for Dealing With Anxiety

Test anxiety is a specific type of anxiety. Symptoms include upset stomach, sweaty palms, tachycardia, trouble concentrating, and a feeling of dread. But there are ways to cope with test anxiety.

- There is no substitute for being well-prepared.

- Practice relaxation techniques.

- Avoid alcohol, excess coffee, caffeine, and any new medications that might sedate you, dull your senses, or make you feel agitated.

- Take a few deep breaths and concentrate on the task at hand.

Focus on Specific Test-Taking Skills

To do well on the exam, you need good test-taking skills in addition to knowledge of the content and ability to use critical thinking.

All Certification Exams Are Multiple Choice

▶ Multiple-choice tests have specific rules for test construction.

▶ A multiple-choice question consists of three parts: the information (or stem), the question, and the four possible answers (one correct and three distracters).

▶ Careful analysis of each part is necessary. Read the entire question before answering.

▶ Practice your test-taking skills by analyzing the practice questions in this book and on the ANCC website.

Analyze the Information Given

▶ Do not assume you have more information than is given.

▶ Do not overanalyze.

▶ Remember, the writer of the question assumes this is all of the information needed to answer the question.

▶ If information is not given, it is not relevant and will not affect the answer.

▶ Do not make the question more complicated than it is.

What Kind of Question Is Asked?

▶ Are you supposed to recall a fact, apply facts to a situation, or understand and differentiate between options?

▷ Read the question thinking about what the writer is asking.

▷ Look for key words or phrases that lead you (see Figure 1–1). These help determine what kind of answer the question requires.

FIGURE 1–1.
EXAMPLES OF KEY WORDS AND PHRASES

▶ avoid	▶ initial	▶ most
▶ best	▶ first	▶ significant
▶ except	▶ contributing to	▶ likely
▶ not	▶ appropriate	▶ of the following
		▶ most consistent with

Read All of the Answers

▶ If you are absolutely certain that answer "a" is correct as you read it, mark it, but read the rest of the question so you do not trick yourself into missing a better answer.

▶ If you are absolutely sure answer "a" is wrong, cross it off or make a note on your scratch paper and continue reading the question.

▶ After reading the entire question, go back, analyze the question, and select the best answer.

▶ Do not jump ahead.

▶ If the question asks you for an assessment, the best answer will be an assessment. Do not be distracted by an intervention that sounds appropriate.

▶ If the question asks you for an intervention, do not answer with an assessment.

▶ When two answer choices sound very good, the best one is usually the least expensive, least invasive way to achieve the goal. For example, if your answer choices include a physical exam maneuver or imaging, the physical exam maneuver is probably the better choice provided it will give the information needed.

▶ If the answers include two options that are the opposite of each other, one of the two is probably the correct answer.

▶ When numeric answers cover a wide range, a number in the middle is more likely to be correct.

▶ Watch out for distracters that are correct but do not answer the question, combine true and false information, or contain a word or phrase that is similar to the correct answer.

▶ Err on the side of caution.

Only One Answer Can Be Correct

▶ When more than one suggested answer is correct, you must identify the one that best answers the question asked.

▶ If you cannot choose between two answers, you have a 50% chance of getting it right if you guess.

Avoid Changing Answers

▶ Change an answer only if you have a compelling reason, such as you remembered something additional, or you understand the question better after rereading it.

▶ People change to a wrong answer more often than to a right answer.

Time Yourself to Complete the Whole Exam

▶ Do not spend a large amount of time on one question.

▶ If you cannot answer a question quickly, mark it and continue the exam.

▶ If time is left at the end, return to the difficult questions.

▶ Make educated guesses by eliminating the obviously wrong answers and choosing a likely answer even if you are not certain.

▶ Trust your instinct.

▶ Answer every question. There is no penalty for a wrong answer.

▶ Occasionally a question will remind you of something that helps you with a question earlier in the test. Look back at that question to see if what you are remembering affects how you would answer that question.

ABOUT THE CERTIFICATION EXAMS

The American Nurses Credentialing Center Computerized Exam

The ANCC examination is given only as a computer exam, and each exam is different. The order of the questions is scrambled for every test, so even if two people are taking the same exam, the questions will be in a different order. The exam consists of 175 multiple-choice questions.

▶ 150 of the 175 questions are part of the test and how you answer will count toward your score; 25 are included to refine questions and will not be scored. You will not know which ones count, so treat all questions the same.

▶ You will need to know how to use a mouse, scroll by either clicking arrows on the scroll bar or using the up and down arrow keys, and perform other basic computer tasks.

▶ The exam does not require computer expertise.

▶ However, if you are not comfortable with using a computer, you should practice using a mouse and computer beforehand so you do not waste time on the mechanics of using the computer.

Know what to expect during the test.

▶ Each ANCC test question is independent of the other questions.

  ▸ For each case study, there is only one question. This means that a correct answer on any question does not depend on the correct answer to any other question.

  ▸ Each question has four possible answers. There are no questions asking for combinations of correct answers (such as "a and c") or multiple-multiples.

▶ You can skip a question and go back to it at the end of the exam.

▶ You cannot mark key words in the question or right or wrong answers. If you want to do this, use the scratch paper.

▶ You will get your results immediately, and a grade report will be provided upon leaving the testing site.

Internet Resources:

▶ ANCC website: www.nursecredentialing.org

▶ ANA Bookstore: www.nursesbooks.org. Catalog of ANA nursing scope and standards publications and other titles that may be listed on your test content outline.

▶ National Guideline Clearinghouse: www.ngc.gov

CHAPTER 2

ORGANIZATIONAL FACTORS

DEFINITIONS

▶ *Culture* refers to the personality of an organization that is determined by various *dynamics* present in the workplace (Andrews & Boyle, 2008).

▶ *Dynamics* are defined as the interacting forces within a group that produce a pattern or process of change, growth, or activity (Merriam-Webster, 2010).

▶ The *purpose* is the reason for the existence of an organization or department.

▶ The words *purpose* and *mission* are often used interchangeably.

▶ A *mission statement* is a statement of purpose that defines the direction and target of an organization's activities.

▶ A *vision* is a statement that describes the desired future of an organization or a department.

▶ *Values* are beliefs and principles that describe the way an organization directs its activities (Abruzzese, 1996).

▶ A *goal* is a long-term organizational target that "states what the department wants to accomplish or become over the next several years" (Anderson, 2013, p. 39).

▶ *Strategic planning* is the process that an organization uses to determine direction, allocate resources, assign responsibilities, and set timelines to achieve realistic strategic goals.

▶ "*Shared governance* can be defined broadly as a nursing management strategy that 'legitimizes' nurses' decision-making control over their professional practice while extending their influence to administrative areas previously controlled by management" (Hess, 1995, p. 14).

ORGANIZATIONAL CULTURE AND DYNAMICS

▶ The vision, mission, values, assumptions, norms, and other factors that influence the dynamics in an organization determine the organizational culture.

▶ Organizational dynamics integrate the analytical work of an organization with the emotional processes of its people. It is influenced by leadership and management styles, number of employees, and geographic locations.

▶ Informal factors such as assumptions and historical norms may also influence the organizational dynamics and, hence, the culture within an organization. For example, employees may maintain and expect behavior that is consistent with well-established traditions about teamwork expectations, meeting behavior, or dress code.

▶ The organizational culture establishes patterns for employees to understand particular events, actions, communications, or situations within the organization. These patterns of understanding help employees manage their behavior as they encounter new experiences in the work environment.

▶ In addition, demographic factors such as size, location, geographic setting, and number of employees also contribute to the organizational culture (Andrews & Boyle, 2008).

▶ Examples of healthcare organizations with distinctly different cultures include

  » 50-bed rural critical access hospital

  » 800-bed tertiary care center in a metropolitan area

  » 500-bed hospital affiliated with a university

  » 45-bed long-term care and hospice facility

  » 200-bed military hospital and clinic

MISSION

▶ The *mission* describes essential functions of an organization or department as well as the reason for its existence (Avillion, 2008).

  » Mission statements clearly and concisely communicate the purpose and direction of an entity's activities.

  » The *vision* is an image or dream of the desired future of an organization.

  » Values (sometimes referred to as philosophy) are beliefs and principles that direct an organization's activities.

▶ A *mission statement* identifies the composition and scope of the department or organization, its reason for existence, and the target audience being served.

▶ The mission statement provides clear direction toward achieving established goals and objectives and an explicit definition to employees (Anderson, 2013).

▶ The mission statement for an education department or program is developed using the organization's mission statement. The departmental mission must reflect the values and beliefs of the department and the organization (Gordon, Habley, & Grites, 1998, as cited in Anderson, 2013; Penn, 2008).

▶ A well-written mission statement for a nursing professional development (NPD) department

  ▸ reflects the organizational mission, values, and vision;

  ▸ focuses on organizational and departmental priorities;

  ▸ serves as the foundation for departmental goals and objectives;

  ▸ and evolves and changes as the organization's priorities change (Anderson, 2013; Avillion, 2008).

▶ The mission statement must be broad, concise, visionary, realistic, and motivational (Anderson, 2013).

▶ Sample mission statement: The staff development department of General Healthcare System supports the mission, vision, and values of the organization by developing and providing educational products and services designed to enhance the quality of patient care. This is accomplished through educational activities intended to increase knowledge and skills of employees in the nursing division. The department is committed to conducting and analyzing research data to identify benchmarks and best practices in the field of nursing professional development.

Vision

▶ A clear and attainable vision creates value. It is inspiring and exciting for employees as they strive individually and collaboratively to achieve the identified future state.

▶ A *vision statement* concisely describes the department's or the organization's desired state in aspirational, inspirational, and measurable terms (Anderson, 2013).

▶ A vision must be precise, realistic, easily understood, and clearly written so that it is meaningful to employees, patients, and other stakeholders (Avillion, 2008).

▶ Sample vision statement: It is the vision of the education and professional development division to be a regional leader in the provision of education programs that focus on excellence in oncology healthcare services and to conduct educational research for the purpose of identifying best practices in continuing education for oncology nurses.

VALUES

▶ The values and beliefs of a department or organization are expressed in its philosophy.

▶ Values serve as the foundational principles that guide the behavior, character, and culture of a department or organization (Anderson, 2013).

▶ Values may be incorporated into mission statements or may supplement a mission statement as a declaration of what is important to the department (Golway, 2009).

▶ Values exert a powerful influence on how each individual chooses to react and behave in specific situations (Andrews & Boyle, 2008).

▶ For employees of a department to live its values, the following must occur:

  ▹ Employees use the established values to guide their work performance, priority-setting, decision-making, and interactions.

  ▹ Rewards and recognition are awarded to employees whose work reflects the departmental values.

  ▹ Recruitment and retention efforts focus on hiring and keeping employees whose work behaviors are congruent with the departmental values (Heathfield, 2007).

▶ Factors that affect nursing professional development may influence the values of an educational department or organization. These factors include:

  ▹ Environment: Patient population, demographics, healthcare delivery systems, cultural variations in staff and patient groups, and setting;

  ▹ Learner characteristics: Learning style, educational background, experience, personal values; and

  ▹ Educational design: Classroom, online, independent study, audio- or teleconference (Kelly-Thomas, 1998).

▶ Consistent values across all levels of an organization result in fewer conflicts and greater commitment by all employees.

▶ Values of the American Nurses Credentialing Center's Accreditation Program include (ANCC, 2013)

  ▹ Process integrity

  ▹ Competence

  ▹ Quality

  ▹ Mentorship

  ▹ Accountability and responsiveness

- Innovation

- Diversity and inclusiveness

- Fiscal responsibility and accountability

- Lifelong learning

- Interprofessional activities

- Collaboration

GOALS

▶ *Goals* are broadly written statements that guide an organization to complete activities that will contribute to achievement of the mission.

▶ Goals for a nursing professional development department must be based on relevant, appropriate organizational goals so that educational efforts contribute to achievement of the organization's goals (Avillion, 2008).

▶ Although goals are derived from the mission and values of the department, they are more concrete and specific to serve as a basis for developing more detailed outcomes for specific programmatic areas.

▶ Because the primary mission of nursing professional development is to provide educational programs and services, departmental goal statements cover programmatic areas such as orientation, continuing education, competency assessment, and in-service.

▶ Goals may focus on the outcomes of programmatic areas in education or on the educational processes used to achieve these outcomes (Kelly-Thomas, 1998).

▶ Goals in the educational process are broad, global statements of the final outcomes to be achieved at the end of the teaching and learning processes.

▶ Educational goals are multidimensional; they incorporate several specific objectives of a learning activity (Bastable, 2008).

▶ The goals of a nursing professional development department change as the needs and priorities of the organization change.

▶ Because goals of a nursing professional development department evolve as the organization evolves, it is important to conduct periodic, systematic reviews to confirm, revise, or update the goals to ensure that they remain consistent with the direction of the organization (Alspach, 1995).

▶ Sample goals for a nursing professional development department:

  ▹ By the end of the fiscal year, 50% of the rehabilitation staff nurses will complete a certification review course in their clinical specialty.

  ▹ Use of the simulation center for emergency response training updates will be implemented in all critical care areas within the next 6 months.

  ▹ The nursing professional development department will reduce printing expenditures by 10% through conversion to electronic communication and documentation.

STRATEGIC PLANNING

▶ *Strategic planning* is the process that an organization uses to determine direction, allocate resources, assign responsibilities, and set timelines to achieve realistic strategic goals.

▶ The strategic planning process is applicable and shared at the unit, departmental, and institutional levels of an organization.

▶ Strategic planning extends 3 to 5 years into the future.

▶ Strategic planning process steps:

  ▹ Conduct a SWOT (strengths, weaknesses, opportunities, threats) analysis.

  ▹ Review and revise mission, vision, and values statements.

  ▹ Identify strategic and operational goals.

  ▹ Establish objectives and strategies to achieve goals.

  ▹ Implement and evaluate effectiveness of strategies and achievement of objectives (Tomey, 2009).

▶ An executive summary is a one- to two-page document that summarizes the key elements of the plan. It

  ▹ Refreshes the memory of the reader concerning the project,

  ▹ Provides a "5-minute" summary, and

  ▹ May be the only section of the plan that gets read (Apeles, 2009).

SHARED GOVERNANCE

Structure

- ▶ Shared governance is more than the current buzzword in nursing. Shared governance has existed in nursing for longer than 30 years, beginning in the 1980s.

- ▶ Shared governance, also known as shared accountability, is a comprehensive approach to management by nurses for nurses and patient care.

- ▶ Shared governance is a decentralized process of decision-making that affords nurses a powerful position in an organization.

- ▶ This approach places decision-making at the point of care by the experts in direct care delivery.

Decision-Making by Nurses

- ▶ In shared governance, unit-based councils (process teams) make decisions to change what is in their control and may make recommendations for matters not in their purview. It requires that participants

  - ▹ Identify the boundaries of the council's influence

  - ▹ Educate nurses on how to

    - ▷ Substantiate the need for change

    - ▷ Determine timing of requests and recommendations

    - ▷ Initiate change

    - ▷ Solicit peer feedback

    - ▷ Collect new data once implementation occurs

    - ▷ Synthesize or analyze data

    - ▷ Interpret data outcomes

    - ▷ Establish time frames for reevaluation

  - ▹ Transforming Care at the Bedside, the Institute for Healthcare Improvement's collaborative quality improvement program, helps staff in unit-based councils determine needs and prioritize them in the resolution process. Nurses make the difference in implementing changes that will improve quality and outcomes.

  - ▹ The clinical specialist or nursing professional development specialist may facilitate council meetings.

  - ▹ Advanced practice nurses may co-chair with a staff nurse or may serve as vice-chair with the staff nurse as chair.

▶ Service-based shared governance councils offer opportunities for nurses from similar units to discuss positive and not-so-positive outcomes they have experienced through their decision-making processes.

  ▶ Best practices, standards of care, and publishable data outcomes have been generated from councils such as these.

  ▶ A manager or director facilitates the process meeting.

  ▶ A manager may serve as vice-chair with the staff nurse as chair.

▶ Shared governance coordinating councils prepare staff nurses to move professionally in the structure and process of the Magnet Model®. The shared governance coordinating council membership structure may differ between institutions. Staff nurse members of the coordinating council may be elected by their peers to be service-based council representatives. These representatives work with the council facilitator, a nursing management member.

  ▶ A two-way flow of communication enables the sharing of accomplishments, issues, concerns, and decisions made at the coordinating council level.

  ▶ Hospital, state, accrediting body, and Magnet Model standards are reflected in the decisions made during the council meetings.

  ▶ Decisions of the coordinating council may assist in changing the standards and practices of patient care related to specific aspects of care delivery and nursing processes.

  ▶ The chief nursing officer (CNO), associate CNO, or divisional director facilitates the meeting.

  ▶ The CNO co-chairs with a staff nurse.

Shared Governance Process

▶ Shared governance is a dynamic process that provides a framework for practice. It

  ▶ Is a continuum

  ▶ Provides a voice for professional nursing

  ▶ Increases participation in operational and policy decision-making

  ▶ Provides collaboration with other colleagues in addressing clinical and administrative challenges

  ▶ Provides collegial relationships with other professionals

  ▶ Has bylaws or constitutions of the shared governance councils that provide substance to the framework

- ▶ Shared governance structural factors include

  - » Education and ongoing training

  - » Coaching and monitoring

  - » Clear structure for decision-making

  - » Assistance in setting realistic goals

  - » Identification of issues for the decision-making process

  - » Pathways for input

  - » Budgeted time for meetings

  - » Staff support for meeting attendance data and information flow process

  - » Supporting roles (e.g., clerical; Ballard, 2010)

- ▶ The essence of shared governance is collaboration or partnership. It establishes structure for creating goal alignments, which begins with the strategic planning goals of the organization. Nursing department goals align with these goals. Emphasis on strategic goal-planning becomes manifest in council goals, whether service-oriented, departmental, or unit-based, culminating with the patient care goals of the individual nurse.

- ▶ Ownership and accountability for the process of decision-making forms the basis for desirable outcomes and requires a shift in:

  - » Lines of authority

  - » Perceptions of professional responsibility

  - » Distribution of power

- ▶ Shared governance literature identifies six dimensions of governance:

  - » Control over professional practice

  - » Influence over organizational resources that support practice

  - » Formal authority granted by the organization

  - » Committee structures that allow participation in decision-making

  - » Access to information about the organization

  - » Ability to set goals and negotiate conflict

▶ The key components are:

  ▹ Practice

  ▹ Quality

  ▹ Education

  ▹ Peer process (Finkelman, 2006)

▶ The process of shared governance requires the nursing professional development specialist and nursing management to work in harmony or the process may break down.

▶ Managers may have the steepest learning curve to navigate.

▶ Accountability and authority are essential for nurses to assume the new role.

▶ Education is planned over time.

  ▹ Definitions

  ▹ Structure and process

  ▹ Anticipated outcome

  ▹ Resource allocation and access to resources

  ▹ Support personnel

  ▹ Frequently asked questions

  ▹ A variety of teaching strategies, with heavy emphasis on simulation

  ▹ An ongoing commitment; times, people, and environment change

▶ Management responsibilities:

  ▹ Remove as many barriers as possible.

  ▹ Promote collaborative environment.

  ▹ Promote open communication.

  ▹ Facilitate decision-making groups.

  ▹ Support decisions made.

  ▹ Facilitate implementation.

  ▹ Start small; work toward great.

  ▹ Recognize and reward successes.

▶ Implications for Magnet® facilities:

  ▹ The 2009 Magnet Model has five component parts that delineate the expected structures and processes of an organization:

    ▷ Transformational leadership

    ▷ Structural empowerment

    ▷ Exemplary professional practice

    ▷ New knowledge, innovation, and implementation

    ▷ Empirical outcomes

▶ All components are influenced by or influence the internal and external healthcare environment.

▶ The major components that relate to shared governance are transformational leadership (focusing on the CNO) and structural empowerment (focusing on the direct care professional nurse).

▶ "Magnet facilities achieve designation due to the practice that is supported by the framework of shared governance, not due to the framework" (Porter O'Grady, 2003, p. 252).

▶ The Index of Professional Nursing Governance (IPNG) was developed in the 1990s and remains a respected measure of professional nursing governance of hospital-based nurses.

  ▹ Measurement tool includes

    ▷ 88-item index

    ▷ The six dimensions of shared governance

      ▹ Professional control

      ▹ Organizational influence

      ▹ Organizational recognition

      ▹ Facilitating attributes

      ▹ Liaison

      ▹ Alignment (Hess, 1998)

Strategies for the Nursing Professional Development Specialist

▶ How can the nursing professional development specialist support the development or maintenance of a shared governance framework?

  ▹ Learn as much as possible about the framework and process.

  ▹ Take the Forum for Shared Governance (www.sharedgovernance.org) free 1-hour course supported by nurse.com.

  ▹ Make yourself indispensable to the process.

    ▹ Ask questions and find answers:

      ▹ What features should be included in the structure?

      ▹ Who needs to be involved in development?

      ▹ Who needs to be involved in maintenance?

      ▹ What is the first priority or focus?

      ▹ How would council members be selected?

      ▹ What information do all staff members need?

      ▹ How do the unit-based and service-based councils integrate with the whole shared governance process?

      ▹ What should be the timeline for development, education, and implementation of the shared governance framework and process? (Newman, 2010)

▶ Create a checklist for designing a shared governance model.

▶ Develop tools to promote council efficiency:

  ▹ Constitution or bylaws

  ▹ Election cycle for membership

  ▹ Minutes tracking form

  ▹ Guidelines for how to run a meeting

▶ Assist in planning how council meetings will be run:

  ▹ Title of council

  ▹ Membership

  ▹ Bylaws or constitution

  ▹ Timing—when meetings will be held and how long they will last

- ▹ Location

- ▹ Voting process

- ▹ Recorder

- ▹ Minutes format

- ▹ Reporting process

▶ Plan, develop, and present educational activities to support the shared governance process.

▶ Become instrumental in the selection or development of a peer review process.

▶ Develop a quantitative research project to study governance. Determine return on investment (ROI).

▶ Promote rewards for and recognition of nurses in the organization.

▶ "The patient care council and the services framework are designed specifically to ensure that 90 percent of the decisions are made at the point of service" (Porter O'Grady, Hawkins, & Parker, 1997, p. 134).

▶ "Since the point of service is the fundamental place of decision making in the organization, it is critical that patient care design facilitate decision making at that point in service" (Porter O'Grady, Hawkins, & Parker, 1997, p. 125).

▶ Direct care nurse–driven decision-making is a strong indicator of excellence in governance. The output of the framework of shared governance leads to excellence in patient care.

Organizational Structure

▶ The organizational structure for nursing professional development departments may be centralized, decentralized, or a combination.

▶ The manager of the nursing professional development work unit may report to an administrator in the nursing department, human resources, or another administrative position within or across sites.

▶ Placement of the nursing professional development staff and work unit within the organizational structure influences and is influenced by the unit's responsibilities and scope.

▶ Other factors that affect the responsibilities and scope of nursing professional development within an organization include size of organization, number of employees, organizational mission, and type of institution (Puetz & Aucoin, 2002).

▶ Nursing professional development may be structured in one of the following ways, each of which has quality advantages and disadvantages:

  ▸ Institution-wide: All educators are in an identified, centralized department responsible for staff education in multiple departments throughout the institution. The work unit may be based in nursing, human resources, education, or another nonclinical department.

    ▷ Advantages: Coordination of resources and required programming, uniform implementation of standards, comprehensive orientation, consistent content and teaching methods, efficient use of staff and support services

    ▷ Disadvantages: May be unaware of or unresponsive to unit needs, lack of coordination or identity with specific areas, potential loss of autonomy or clinical skills of educators

  ▸ Nursing department: Department or division responsible for education of nursing department staff. Some NPD specialists may be centralized to manage general educational activities, while others are unit- or service line–based to manage unit-specific educational activities. NPD specialists who are decentralized may be full-time in education or may have patient care responsibilities in addition to the educational role.

    ▷ Advantages: Easier identification of unit educational needs, flexibility and timeliness in providing educational activities, educational leadership and involvement in departments, increased opportunity for feedback, educators seen as clinical experts

    ▷ Disadvantages: Duplication of education and staff effort, inconsistent education content and teaching methods, ineffective or inefficient coordination, lack of support services, NPD specialists may be used for service

  ▸ Combination of institution-wide and nursing department: Uses portion of both centralized and decentralized structures to manage and deliver education.

    ▷ Advantages: Identification of and timely response to unit needs, use of clinical experts for unit-based educational activities, coordination reduces duplication and inappropriate use of resources, availability of support services, collegial support for educators

    ▷ Disadvantages: Potential increased staffing and costs of managing both structures, NPD specialists may lose sight of overall staff development goals (Alspach, 1995; Brunt, 1998; Hood, 2002)

» Cooperative or consortium: Collaborative effort between two or more organizations (e.g., hospital, college or university, long-term-care facility) in which professional development educators share responsibilities for staff education; may include nursing and nonnursing roles

  ▷ Advantage: Ability to provide more and higher-quality programs at a lower cost

  ▷ Disadvantage: Requires collaboration and shared planning for consensus on products, facilities, and resources (Brunt, 1998)

REFERENCES

Abruzzese, R. S. (Ed.). (1996). *Nursing staff development: Strategies for success*. St. Louis, MO: Mosby.

Alspach, J. G. (1995). *The educational process in nursing staff development*. St. Louis, MO: Mosby.

American Nurses Credentialing Center. (2013). 2013 *ANCC primary accreditation application manual for providers and approvers*. Silver Spring, MD: Author.

Anderson, D. A. (2013). Mission, vision and strategic planning in nursing professional development. In S. L. Bruce (Ed.), *Core curriculum for nursing professional development* (4th ed., pp. 31–45). Chicago: Association for Nursing Professional Development.

Andrews, M. M., & Boyle, J. S. (2008). *Transcultural concepts in nursing care* (5th ed.). Philadelphia: Lippincott Williams & Wilkins.

Apeles, N. C. (2009). Business and financial aspects of staff development. In S. Bruce (Ed.), *Core curriculum for staff development* (3rd ed.). Pensacola, FL: National Nursing Staff Development Organization.

Avillion, A. E. (2008). *A practical guide to staff development: Evidence-based tools and techniques for effective education* (2nd ed.). Marblehead, MA: HCPro.

Ballard, N. (2010). Factors associated with success and breakdown of shared governance. *Journal of Nursing Administration, 40*(10), 411–416.

Bastable, S. B. (2008). *Nurse as educator: Principles of teaching and learning for nursing practice*. Boston: Jones & Bartlett.

Brunt, B. A. (1998). Structure and process: New models of nursing and clinical staff development. In K. J. Kelly-Thomas (Ed.), *Clinical and nursing staff development: Current competence, future focus* (2nd ed., pp. 25–53). Philadelphia: Lippincott Williams & Wilkins.

Dynamics. (2010). *Merriam-Webster online dictionary*. Retrieved from http://www.merriam-webster.com/dictionary/dynamics

Finkleman, A. W. (2006). *Leadership and management in nursing*. Upper Saddle River, NJ: Pearson Education.

Golway, M. M. (2009). Purpose, philosophy, and objectives. In S. L. Bruce (Ed.), *Core curriculum for staff development* (3rd ed., pp. 21–32). Pensacola, FL: National Nursing Staff Development Organization.

Heathfield, S. (2007). Build a strategic framework through strategic planning. *About.com: Money > human resources*. Retrieved from http://humanresources.about.com/cs/strategicplanning1/a/strategicplan.htm

Hess, R. (1995). Shared governance: Nursing's 20th-century Tower of Babel. *Journal of Nursing Administration, 25*(5), 14–17.

Hess, R. (1998). Measuring nursing governance. *Nursing Research, 47*(1), 35–42.

Hood., A. W. (2002). Factors that affect the educator's role. In K. L. O'Shea (Ed.), *Staff development nursing secrets* (pp. 17–25). Philadelphia: Lippincott.

Kelly-Thomas, K. J. (1998). *Clinical and nursing staff development: Current competence, future focus* (2nd ed.). Philadelphia: Lippincott.

Newman, K. P. (2010). Transforming organizational culture through nursing shared governance. *Nursing Clinics of North America, 46*(1), 45–58.

Penn, B. K. (2008). *Mastering the teaching role: A guide for nurse educators.* Philadelphia: F. A. Davis.

Porter O'Grady, T. (2003). Researching shared governance, futility in focus. *Journal of Nursing Administration, 33*(4), 251–252.

Porter O'Grady, T., Hawkins, M., & Parker, M. (1997). *Whole-systems shared governance: Architecture for integration.* Gaithersburg, MD: Aspen.

Puetz, B. E., & Aucoin, J. W. (2002). *Conversations in nursing professional development.* Pensacola, FL: Pohl.

Tomey, A. M. (2009). *Guide to nursing management and leadership* (8th ed.). St. Louis, MO: Elsevier.

CHAPTER 3

PRINCIPLES OF EDUCATION

BACKGROUND

▶ *Teaching* is an art and science in which structured, sequenced information and experiences are transmitted to produce learning.

▶ *Learning* occurs when a person changes behavior, mental processing, or emotional functioning as a result of exposure to new knowledge or experience (Braungart & Braungart, 2008).

▶ *Andragogy* is the art and science of teaching adults.

▶ Fundamental principles that guide the planning, implementation, and evaluation of adult education:

   ▸ Lifelong learning is the learner's responsibility.

   ▸ Lifelong learning is essential to maintain competence.

   ▸ Competence is critical to the delivery of quality, appropriate patient care.

   ▸ The nursing professional development specialist acts as a facilitator who actively partners with the learner during educational activities.

   ▸ The nursing professional development specialist is responsible for considering adult learning principles in planning and implementing educational activities that meet the needs of the organization and its employees.

   ▸ Various formats are used to deliver educational activities to accommodate the diverse learning styles, learning needs, and characteristics of nurse populations.

   ▸ The nursing professional development specialist is responsible for evaluating progress toward the attainment of outcomes (American Nurses Association, 2010).

PRINCIPLES OF ADULT EDUCATION

▶ Adults need a reason for learning.

  ▷ Adults want to know from a personal perspective why it is important to attend an educational activity.

  ▷ Communicating evidence that supports the need for an educational program is essential. Adults have the right and responsibility to know the rationale for attending educational activities.

▶ Adults are self-directed learners responsible for their own learning.

  ▷ Self-direction in adults stems from a desire to have control over what they learn and how they learn it.

  ▷ Adults participate in the planning, implementation, and evaluation of educational activities.

  ▷ Adults participate in assessing educational needs.

▶ Adults bring varied life experiences to learning situations.

  ▷ Life experiences may enhance learning even if they do not directly relate to the program topic.

  ▷ Adult learners should be encouraged to share their life experiences if they are willing to do so.

  ▷ The nursing professional development educator facilitates learning by helping learners apply their personal experiences to enhance the learning process.

▶ Adults are life-oriented learners. They focus on obtaining knowledge and skills that will help them in their daily lives.

  ▷ Adults need to understand how specific knowledge, skills, and behaviors will benefit them in job performance, interpersonal interactions, and professional development.

  ▷ Adults become impatient if they are forced to participate in educational activities that they believe are not purposeful or beneficial to work or their personal lives.

  ▷ Adults approach education from a task-, problem-, or life-oriented perspective.

▶ Adults respond to both intrinsic and extrinsic motivators.

  ▷ Motivators are factors perceived to be of benefit to the learner.

  ▷ Examples of extrinsic motivators include salary increases, promotions, improved working conditions, and public recognition.

» Examples of intrinsic motivators include increased self-esteem, ability to enhance interpersonal relationships, and enhanced job satisfaction.

» Adults are more responsive to intrinsic motivators. Connecting educational program purpose to the adult learner's intrinsic motivators increases learning.

» Nursing professional development educators must consider internal and external motivators when planning learning activities (Avillion, 2008).

LEARNING THEORIES

Behaviorism

▶ "Learning is viewed as a change in behavior or a change in response primarily due to environmental factors" (Schunk, 2012, as cited in Ellis, 2013, p. 50).

▶ Behavioral theory focuses on overt, measurable, observable behavior.

▶ Also called the S-R mode of learning, behavioral theory suggests that learning occurs in response to altered stimulus conditions in the environment or reinforcement after a response.

▶ Behavioral theory applies the principles of respondent conditioning (responses are conditioned or unconditioned reflexes) and operant conditioning (desired behavior is reinforced to encourage the frequency of a desired response) to the learning situation.

▶ Transfer of learning occurs through repeated practice and consistent, immediate reinforcement.

▶ The educator's role is to arrange the environment, including the reinforcement, to produce desired behavior change and eliminate undesirable behavior (Vandeveer, 2009).

Cognitive Learning Theory

▶ Cognitive learning theory states that learning is a highly active process directed by the learner, who uses cognitive skills to acquire and apply new information.

▶ Cognitive learning theory focuses on reorganizing information into new insights or understanding.

▶ Goals and expectations within the individual create disequilibrium, which produces the motivation for learning.

▶ The learner controls transfer of learning through information processing and application.

▶ Recognizing the learners' past experiences, perceptions, ways of processing information, and social influences that affect any learning situation is the focus of the educator.

▶ The educator's role is to consider available information about the learners when organizing and presenting the educational content (Braungart & Braungart, 2008; Vandeveer, 2009).

Humanism

▶ Humanistic learning theory is based on the belief that each person is unique, autonomous, and wants to grow in a positive way.

▶ According to this theory, self-direction and individual life experiences are essential to the process of learning.

▶ Self-evaluation, internal motivation, self-concept, and self-discovery are all important to the humanistic learning process.

▶ "Learning has an impact on behavior, attitudes and personality of the learner" (Ellis, 2013, p. 51).

▶ The educator's role is to facilitate learning, not to serve as the source of all information (Braungart & Braungart, 2008; Vandeveer, 2009).

Multiple Intelligences Theory

▶ Multiple intelligences theory, based on the work of Howard Gardner, proposes that each individual possesses a unique profile of eight intelligences that forms the basis for learning throughout life.

▶ This theory focuses on biopsychosocial potentials that work together to promote individual learning and development, problem-solving, and interaction with the environment.

▶ The intelligences that work together to produce learning are bodily-kinesthetic, spatial, linguistic, logical-mathematical, musical, interpersonal, intrapersonal, and naturalist. Existential intelligence, moral intelligence, and spiritual intelligence are three other areas that Gardner suggested be studied further before adding them to the list of intelligences.

▶ Different people have different strengths and learn in different ways.

▶ The educator's role is to use knowledge of learners' profiles or the intelligences themselves to design meaningful learning experiences (Lowenstein & Bradshaw, 2001; Vandeveer, 2009).

CHARACTERISTICS OF ADULT LEARNERS

▶ Educators of adults have a responsibility to consider the characteristics of adult learners in planning, implementing, and evaluating learning experiences (Alspach, 1995; Bastable, 2008; Ellis, 2013; Kelly-Thomas, 1998).

▶ Because adults are heterogeneous learners, educators will

   » Involve learners in determining their own learning needs and how to meet them.

   » Expect and encourage differences of opinion and meaning.

   » Respect the unique perspective and background of each learner.

▶ Because adults have multiple responsibilities, educators will

   » Recognize that other responsibilities may interfere with readiness, participation, or learning achievement.

   » Provide flexibility in scheduling, teaching strategies, and options for learning to make education convenient for adults.

   » Provide opportunities for adults to participate actively in all phases of the educational experience.

▶ Because adults bring various life and work backgrounds to the current educational experience, educators will

   » Assess past experiences and incorporate them into the educational activity.

   » Value the knowledge and skills that learners bring from their backgrounds to an educational environment.

   » Use teaching strategies that build on past experiences.

   » Emphasize the relationship between past experiences and present content to encourage transfer of learning.

▶ Because adults may be less flexible than children as learners, educators will

   » Be open-minded and adaptable in designing educational activities.

   » Help learners integrate new concepts with previous beliefs and perspectives.

   » Give learners time to work through new information, consider how new concepts fit, and reach their own conclusions.

- Because adults may have negative past learning experiences, educators will
    - Provide frequent positive reinforcement.
    - Create a learning climate that is conducive to a positive educational experience.
    - Show confidence in the learner's abilities to acquire the necessary knowledge and skills to change behavior.
    - Give learners positive or constructive feedback about performance.
  - Because adults are voluntary learners, educators will:
    - Assess the motivational factors that influence learner participation in the educational activity.
    - Maintain realistic expectations of learners based on their motivation for attending the educational activity.
    - Identify and respond to behavioral cues that suggest that the learner's needs are not being met.
- Adults are problem-centered learners who respond to educators who
    - Identify and meet the learner's priority needs.
    - Focus the educational content on concrete essentials that learners can apply to their own situations.
    - Use a problem-centered approach that relates educational content to real-life situations.
- Educators who recognize that adults are knowledgeable learners will
    - Approach learners as peers who are knowledgeable colleagues.
    - Display mutual respect and a sense of collegiality in interactions with learners.
    - Encourage learners to experiment and learn from their mistakes when possible, but be available to support learners when needed.
    - Provide helpful, useful, clear information using realistic scenarios to illustrate content.
- Because most adults are self-directed in their learning, educators will
    - Provide opportunities for learners to use their own goals and expectations to evaluate the effectiveness of the educational activity.
    - Respond to evaluation feedback to provide additional educational support or make changes in future educational activities.

▶ Because adults of different ages need varying degrees of support in learning, educators will

   ▹ Create a learning environment (e.g., seating, ventilation, lighting, acoustics) that is comfortable and conducive to learning for people with varied physical, mental, emotional, and social capabilities.

   ▹ Check in with learners often to adjust the pace of learning activities or provide support as needed.

   ▹ Arrange coverage of content so that the most complex or challenging material is addressed when learners are at peak performance (Alspach, 1995; Fischer, 2009).

LEARNING STYLES

▶ Learning style preferences refer to the ways in which learners prefer to approach learning as well as the conditions under which they learn most effectively and efficiently (Alspach, 1995; Kitchie, 2008).

▶ Learning style may be influenced over time by factors such as the environment, life experiences, job changes and demands, and personality traits.

▶ Learning is more likely to occur at educational activities that are designed to correspond with the learning styles of the audience (Kitchie, 2008).

Six Learning Style Principles

1. Both the educator's teaching style and the learner's learning style can be identified.

2. Educators must avoid relying on teaching methods and tools that fit their own preferred styles.

3. Educators are most helpful when they assist learners to identify their own learning style preferences and pursue educational activities that match those preferences.

4. Learners should have the chance to learn using their preferred learning style.

5. Learners should be encouraged to take advantage of opportunities to expand their learning style preferences.

6. Educators can develop educational activities that support each learning style (Kitchie, 2008).

Learning Style Inventories

▶ A number of instruments can be used to measure learning styles and preferences.

▶ "Knowing and understanding their learning style or preference may help the learner learn and study more effectively" (Smith, 2013, p. 238).

Kolb's Experiential Learning Model

▶ Kolb's Experiential Learning Model is based on the premise that adults refine their approaches to learning over time as they perceive and process information. Influencing factors include past experiences, current environmental demands, and heredity. This model emphasizes the way meaning is attached to experience, not just the collection of experiences.

▶ Kolb's model describes four styles of learning that are reflective of two dimensions: perception and processing.

▶ Four modes of learning are identified as steps in the learning cycle: concrete experience (feeling), reflective observation (watching), abstract conceptualization (thinking), and active experimentation (doing).

▶ Based on the learner's strengths in perception and processing through the four modes of learning, Kolb described these four learning styles:

1. *Diverger:* The learner emphasizes concrete experience and reflective observation (feeling and watching). These learners are sensitive and interested in people.

2. *Assimilator:* The learner combines reflective observation and abstract conceptualization (watching and thinking). These learners focus on ideas and concepts.

3. *Converger:* The learner integrates abstract conceptualization and active experimentation (thinking and doing). These learners excel at deductive reasoning to address specific problems or find the best solutions.

4. *Accommodator:* The learner uses active experimentation and concrete experience (doing and feeling). These learners are oriented to facts and use intuitive, trial-and-error methods (Kolb, 1984).

Sensory Learning

▶ Sensory learning style theories reflect the belief that learners have preferences for the senses that they find most effective in processing information.

▶ *Visual learners* learn best through visual stimuli in an otherwise passive environment. These learners are attracted to images, handouts, colorful presentations, and dialogue with imagery.

▶ *Auditory learners* prefer to learn through the spoken word. These learners prefer audiotapes, lectures, or interactive dialogue and respond well to verbal directions.

▶ *Aural learners* like to learn through sound and music. These learners prefer information within a musical context or background.

▶ *Verbal learners* use a combination of the written and spoken word to learn most effectively. These learners like to learn through debates, concept papers, and simulation.

▶ *Kinesthetic learners* learn through hands-on involvement and physical activities. These learners learn most effectively through skill demonstrations, simulation, and experiential activities.

▶ The VARK (Visual-Auditory-Read/Write-Kinesthetic) is one tool that measures sensory learning styles (Avillion, 2008; Fischer, 2009; Kitchie, 2008).

Benner's Novice to Expert Model

▶ Benner's Novice to Expert Model of Skill Acquisition describes how nurses acquire practice skills and knowledge.

▶ According to this model, skill acquisition is dependent on the learner's knowledge and experience over time.

▶ The five levels of nursing practice are:

1. *Novice* (new student nurse): The learner has no background or experience.

2. *Advanced beginner* (graduate nurse): The learner has some experience and needs extensive experiences.

3. *Competent* (2 to 3 years): The learner has a sense of mastery and is able to perform adequately on a day-to-day basis unless major variations occur.

4. *Proficient:* The learner perceives global aspects of situations, recognizes variations, and knows how to modify plans appropriately.

5. *Expert:* The learner intuitively grasps each situation and problem-solves creatively and effectively (Benner, Tanner, & Chesla, 1996, as cited in Ellis, 2013).

VARIATIONS IN LEARNER CHARACTERISTICS

Generational Differences

▶ Currently, the workforce is composed of four generations, each with its own set of characteristics, values, and preferences.

▶ Since educators often deal with audiences that include people from all four generations, a variety of activities can be used to address some of the needs and preferences of each generation.

▶ *Veterans* (born between 1925 and 1945) are products of the Great Depression and World War II. Veterans want recognition for their extensive knowledge and experience. They value tradition, hard work, and adherence to rules. As learners, veterans respect educators as authority figures and prefer formal learning environments and experiences (Avillion, 2008; Gallo, 2011, as cited in Engvall, 2013).

▶ *Baby Boomers* (born between 1946 and 1964) are the result of the healthy postwar economy, civil rights movement, and Vietnam War. They enjoy learning, have a passion to achieve success, and want to make a difference in the world. Baby boomers value teamwork and personal gratification in the workplace. As learners, baby boomers respond best when treated as equals, life experiences are incorporated in learning, and team activities are used (Avillion, 2011, as cited in Engvall, 2013).

▶ *Generation Xers* (born between 1965 and 1980) are often referred to as the "latch-key generation." Their values were shaped by "massive corporate layoffs, technological advances, and increased divorce rates" (Gallo, 2010, as cited in Engvall, 2013, p. 93). They value work–life balance, flexibility, and loyalty to self. As learners, Gen Xers prefer self-directed learning on their terms and stimulating visual or live activities that are fun (Avillion, 2011, as cited in Engvall, 2013).

▶ *Generation Yers* (born between 1981 and 2001) have grown up in a technological era, are globally oriented, and are comfortable with diversity. They are highly motivated and recognize that knowledge and skills increase their job marketability. This is important because they have little company loyalty. As learners, Gen Yers enjoy varied educational strategies and opportunities for creative, interactive exercises (Avillion, 2011; Gallo, 2011 as cited in Engvall, 2013).

Cultural Diversity

▶ Because cultural diversity is a valued social and demographic part of society, nursing professional development educators work with learners from a variety of cultures.

▶ *Culture* is defined as the socially transmitted behavioral patterns, arts, beliefs, values, customs, and other characteristics of a group that guide their worldview and actions.

▶ "Cultural and linguistic competence is a set of congruent behaviors, attitudes, and policies that come together in a system, agency, or among professionals that enables effective work in cross-cultural situations." (Office of Minority Health, 2007, as cited in Engvall, 2013, p. 14.)

▶ *Acculturation* refers to the process of learning another culture and modifying one's own behavior following exposure to that culture.

▶ *Assimilation* is the process in which people from a nondominant culture adopt the behaviors and attitudes of the dominant culture (Husting, 2009).

▶ The cultural values and beliefs of learners influence the educational process and learning outcomes because they affect the learner's thinking, decisions, and actions (Husting, 2009).

▶ Cultural factors to consider in planning, implementing, and evaluating educational activities include verbal and nonverbal communication patterns and barriers; learning style preferences; beliefs and values; gender, interpersonal, and social roles; and time orientation (Andrews, 2008).

REFERENCES

Alspach, J. G. (1995). *The educational process in nursing staff development*. St. Louis, MO: Mosby.

American Nurses Association and National Nursing Staff Development Organization. (2010). *Nursing professional development: Scope and standards of practice*. Silver Spring, MD: Nursesbooks.org.

Andrews, M. M. (2008). Cultural diversity in the health care workforce. In M. M. Andrews & J. S. Boyle (Eds.), *Transcultural concepts in nursing care* (5th ed., pp. 297–326). Philadelphia: Lippincott Williams & Wilkins.

Avillion, A. E. (2008). *A practical guide to staff development: Evidence-based tools and techniques for effective education* (2nd ed.). Marblehead, MA: HCPro.

Bastable, S. B. (2008). *Nurse as educator: Principles of teaching and learning for nursing practice*. Boston: Jones & Bartlett.

Braungart, M. M., & Braungart, R. G. (2008). Applying learning theories to healthcare practice. In S. B. Bastable (Ed.), *Nurse as educator: Principles of teaching and learning for nursing practice* (3rd ed., pp. 51–89). Boston: Jones & Bartlett.

Ellis, N. F. (2013). Principles of adult learning. In S. L. Bruce (Ed.), *Core curriculum for nursing professional development* (4th ed., p. 47–87). Chicago: Association for Nursing Professional Development.

Engvall, J. C. (2013). Generational differences. In S. L. Bruce (Ed.), *Core curriculum for nursing professional development* (4th ed., pp. 89–105). Chicago: Association for Nursing Professional Development.

Fischer, K. J. (2009). Teaching learning methodologies. In S. L. Bruce (Ed.), *Core curriculum for staff development* (3rd ed., pp. 223–250). Pensacola, FL: National Nursing Staff Development Organization.

Garbutt, S. J. (2013). Cultural diversity awareness: Implications for the nursing professional development specialist. In S. L. Bruce (Ed.), *Core curriculum for nursing professional development* (4th ed., pp. 107–117). Chicago: Association for Nursing Professional Development.

Husting, P. M. (2009). Cultural diversity and competence. In S. L. Bruce (Ed.), *Core curriculum for staff development* (3rd ed., pp. 181–193). Pensacola, FL: National Nursing Staff Development Organization.

Kelly-Thomas, K. J. (1998). *Clinical and nursing staff development: Current competence, future focus* (2nd ed.). Philadelphia: Lippincott.

Kitchie, S. (2008). Determinants of learning. In S. B. Bastable (Ed.), *Nurse as educator: Principles of teaching and learning for nursing practice* (3rd ed., pp. 93–145). Boston: Jones & Bartlett.

Kolb, D. A. (1984). *Experiential learning: Experience as the source of learning and development.* Englewood Cliffs, NJ: Prentice-Hall.

Lowenstein, A. J., & Bradshaw, M. J. (2001). *Fuszard's innovative teaching strategies in nursing* (3rd ed.). Gaithersburg, MD: Aspen.

Smith, C. M. (2013). Teaching learning methodologies. In S. L. Bruce (Ed.), *Core curriculum for nursing professional development* (4th ed., pp. 231–288). Chicago: Association for Nursing Professional Development.

Vandeveer, M. (2009). From teaching to learning: Theoretical foundations. In D. M. Billings & J. A. Halstead. (Eds.), *Teaching in nursing: A guide for faculty* (3rd ed., pp. 189–226). St. Louis, MO: Saunders.

CHAPTER 4

DOMAINS OF LEARNING

BACKGROUND

▶ Benjamin Bloom and other experts in educational psychology developed and published a taxonomy of educational objectives in 1956.

▶ Bloom's taxonomy is easy to understand and implement and, therefore, is widely used in the development, implementation, and evaluation of educational activities.

▶ The taxonomy provides a systematic, practical tool for educators to determine educational objectives based on levels of behavior in the learning process.

▶ The taxonomy is divided into three major classifications or domains of learning: cognitive, affective, and psychomotor (Bastable & Doody, 2008; Kelly-Thomas, 1998; Penn, 2008).

▶ Each classification is subdivided into specific hierarchical categories that reflect simple to complex desired outcomes.

▶ Achievement of complex outcomes is based on the successful integration of simple outcomes to form new behaviors.

▶ Although the domains of learning are classified as separate entities, they are actually interdependent domains that learners may experience simultaneously (e.g., thinking processes influence psychomotor performance; adopted values affect thinking processes; Scheckel, 2009).

▶ Educators must consider the interdependence of the domains of learning when planning educational objectives and activities.

▶ The implementation of a taxonomy based on domains of learning makes it possible for educators and learners to clearly and consistently delineate desired learning outcomes.

▶ Specific verbs, such as "demonstrate," appear in more than one domain of learning. When developing objective statements, both the verb and the content area for which performance is directed specify the learning domain and level.

▶ During the 1990s, a group of cognitive psychologists led by Lorin Anderson updated the taxonomy by renaming and reordering the categories in the cognitive domain (Armstrong, 2009; Clark, 2009; Overbaugh & Schultz, 2010).

▶ Some educators have revised the terminology of Bloom's taxonomy to knowledge (cognitive), skills (psychomotor), and attitude (affective), also referred to as KSA (McManus, 2009).

▶ Goal of critical thinking is to develop reflective analysis and encourage others to reflect critically on the situation.

RELEVANCE TO NURSING PROFESSIONAL DEVELOPMENT PRACTICE

▶ According to the American Nurses Association (2010, p. 14), "learning activity content is individualized to the target audience, the resources available, and the domains of learning."

▶ The taxonomy serves as the foundation for writing measurable learning objectives that clearly identify the desired outcomes of the learning process.

▶ Appropriate learning objectives facilitate the selection of teaching strategies and identification of resources needed for successful completion of learning activities.

▶ Measurable learning objectives facilitate the evaluation process by clearly describing expected learning outcomes.

COGNITIVE DOMAIN

▶ The cognitive domain (ways of knowing) refers to the development of intellectual skills or thinking processes.

▶ Learning in the cognitive domain involves the acquisition of facts and knowledge and making use of that knowledge.

▶ The cognitive domain includes six levels of behaviors. The levels, listed in order from simplest to most complex, are *knowledge, comprehension, application, analysis, synthesis*, and *evaluation*.

▶ Behaviors at each level must be mastered before progressing to the next higher level of behaviors (Hardigan, Cohen, & Hagen, 2006; Scheckel, 2009).

▶ *Knowledge*-level objectives involve the recognition or recall of basic facts or information.

> ▸ Verbs that measure knowledge are *define, recall, identify, list, remember,* and *state.*

> ▸ Example: After attending this program, the learner will list the signs and symptoms of myasthenia gravis.

▶ Objectives that measure the *comprehension* level reflect the ability of the learner to interpret the meaning of knowledge and understand instructions or directions.

> ▸ Verbs used to measure *comprehension* include *describe, explain, locate,* and *estimate.*

> ▸ Example: After completing this learning module, the learner will explain the pathophysiology of respiratory acidosis, respiratory alkalosis, metabolic acidosis, and metabolic alkalosis.

▶ Objectives for the next level of behavior, *application,* refer to the use of an acquired concept in a specific situation.

> ▸ Verbs that measure application include differentiate, apply, use, prepare, and demonstrate.

> ▸ Example: Following this learning lab session, the learner will use the standard algorithm for fluid replacement needs to calculate fluid administration amounts for a patient undergoing a surgical procedure.

▶ The fourth level of cognitive behavior, *analysis,* involves separation of concepts or information into parts and determining the relationships among the parts.

> ▸ Verbs that may be used to measure analysis are *analyze, differentiate, diagram, discriminate,* and *separate.*

> ▸ Example: At the conclusion of this learning activity, the learner will analyze the effectiveness of a new skincare product on wounds.

▶ The next level, *synthesis,* refers to the creation of new knowledge or meaning by combining diverse concepts and elements.

> ▸ Verbs that may be used to measure synthesis include *create, combine, design, plan, propose,* and *revise.*

> ▸ Example: After attending this educational seminar, the learner will create a clinical orientation plan for a novice RN.

- ▶ The highest level of cognitive behavior, evaluation, involves making value judgments about situations, ideas, or materials.

    - » Verbs that may be used to measure the evaluation level include *judge, compare, critique, defend,* and *appraise.*

    - » Example: After participation in this simulation exercise, the learner will critique the performance of team members in an emergency situation (Clark, 2009; Hardigan, Cohen, & Hagen, 2006; McManus, 2009).

- ▶ Methods commonly used to promote learning in the cognitive domain include lecture, individualized instruction (e.g., preceptorship, mentorship, skills training) and independent study activities (e.g., web-based learning, journaling, learning modules; Bastable & Doody, 2008; McManus, 2009).

AFFECTIVE DOMAIN

- ▶ The affective domain (ways of feeling) refers to the way learners deal with emotional aspects or feelings associated with learning.

- ▶ Learning in the affective domain involves internalization or commitment to feelings, values, beliefs, interests, and attitudes.

- ▶ The affective domain includes five categories of behaviors that specify the depth of the learner's emotional responses. The levels, listed in order from simplest to most complex, are *receiving phenomena, responding to phenomena, valuing, organization,* and *characterization of values* (Krathwohl, Bloom, & Masia, 1964, pp. 124–125, as cited in McManus & Maloney, 2013).

- ▶ Behaviors at each level build on previous levels as the learner internalizes feelings, leading to personal growth and a shift from an external to an internal locus of control (Scheckel, 2009).

- ▶ Objectives at the *receiving phenomena* level describe the learner's awareness or willingness to attend to data or receive a stimulus.

    - » Verbs that measure receiving phenomena include *listen, share, accept, select, describe,* and *reply.*

    - » Example: After attending a cultural diversity workshop, the learner will share personal perspectives about cultural influences in the workplace.

▶ The second level of the affective domain, *responding to phenomena*, is addressed by objectives that reflect active learner participation and involvement in a particular situation or phenomenon.

  ▹ Responding to phenomena is measured using verbs such as *participate, state, share, recite develop, interpret,* and *select.*

  ▹ Example: On completion of this learning module, the learner will participate in a debate about the significance of ethical principles in a clinical nursing situation.

▶ *Valuing,* the next level, is based on internal values and beliefs that are exhibited in behaviors and responses. Objectives for valuing reflect the behaviors and responses that demonstrate the worth or value a person attaches to an object, behavior, situation, or phenomenon.

  ▹ Verbs that may be used to assess valuing include *demonstrate, volunteer, support, commit,* and *assume responsibility.*

  ▹ Example: After attending this experiential learning workshop, the learner will demonstrate effective use of debriefing skills to promote learning through simulation.

▶ The next level of the affective domain, *organization,* involves prioritizing values and placing them in a hierarchy of importance to create a unique value system.

  ▹ Verbs that may be used to measure organization are *select, challenge, debate, defend, recommend,* and *prioritize.*

  ▹ Example: After participating in this seminar, the learner will challenge barriers to practice for advanced practice nurses.

▶ At the highest level of the affective domain, *characterization* by a value, the learner integrates a value system that guides the learner's behavior.

  ▹ Characterization by a value is measured using verbs such as *adhere, influence, question, synthesize,* and *verify.*

  ▹ Example: Upon successful completion of this course, the learner will adhere to the ethical code for nurses in daily practice (Bastable & Doody, 2008; Hardigan, Cohen, & Hagen, 2006; McManus, 2009).

▶ Effective teaching strategies to promote learning in the affective domain include high levels of learner involvement that encourage self-exploration (e.g., questioning, games, debate, simulation, role play; Bradshaw & Lowenstein, 2010, as cited in McManus & Maloney, 2013).

PSYCHOMOTOR DOMAIN

▶ The psychomotor domain (ways of doing) refers to physical movement, coordination, and motor skills.

▶ Learning in the psychomotor domain involves acquiring gross and fine motor abilities and neuromuscular coordination to perform increasingly complex actions.

▶ Development of psychomotor skills requires practice and is measured in terms of speed, precision, distance, procedures, or techniques.

▶ The psychomotor domain includes five categories of behaviors. The levels, listed in order from simplest to most complex, are *imitation, manipulation, precision, articulation,* and *naturalization.*

▶ At the most basic level, imitation, objectives refer to the ability to replicate actions with allowance for some weakness and inconsistency in completing the action. Time and speed required are based on learner abilities.

  » Verbs used to measure imitation include *choose, follow, select, describe, identify,* and *display.*

  » Example: After reviewing this video, the learner will select the steps necessary to connect the portable oxygen for patient transport.

▶ Objectives at the second level of the psychomotor domain, *manipulation,* relate to the ability to follow directions to perform specific psychomotor skills after instruction and practice. Coordination, speed, and time required to complete the task may vary.

  » Manipulation may be assessed using verbs such as *show, perform, explain, adhere,* and *provide.*

  » Example: Following a practice session in the skills lab, the learner will perform the procedural steps in medication administration.

▶ Objectives at the next level, *precision,* reflect that actions are carried out in a logical sequence with well-coordinated movements and few noncritical errors. Although coordination is evident at this level, time and speed required for completion are still variable.

  » Verbs that can be used to measure precision include *demonstrate, assemble, organize, fix,* and *construct.*

  » Example: After completing the training module on wound care, the learner will demonstrate wound-care techniques in the clinical setting according to hospital procedure.

▶ The fourth level of the psychomotor domain is *articulation*. Objectives at this level refer to coordinated actions that are completed in a logical sequence with minimal errors. Coordination, time, and speed required are all within reasonable expectations.

  ▸ Verbs that measure articulation include *use, complete, operate, design,* and *originate.*

  ▸ Example: After completing a course and clinical experience on physical assessment techniques, the learner will complete a respiratory assessment using auscultation, palpation, and percussion skills.

▶ At the highest level of the psychomotor domain, *naturalization*, objectives describe actions that are completed automatically, virtually error-free, with coordinated movements and consistent performance.

  ▸ Verbs used to measure naturalization include *adapt, demonstrate, discriminate, create, manipulate,* and *form.*

  ▸ Example: After successfully completing the requirements for a clinical practicum, the learner will demonstrate proficiency in management of the discharge planning process (Huitt, 2003; McManus, 2009; Scheckel, 2009).

▶ Teaching methods that may be effectively used for psychomotor skills include return demonstration, supervised clinical practice, simulation, and other experiential learning activities.

CRITICAL THINKING FRAMEWORK

▶ Purposeful, goal-directed thinking that involves seeking and weighing alternatives and selecting the best method to meet the desired outcome (Luckowski, 2009)

▶ Required in nursing curricula by the American Association of Colleges of Nursing and the National League for Nursing Accrediting Commission (Walsh and Seldomridge, 2006)

▶ Goal of critical thinking is to develop reflective analysis and encourage others to reflect critically on the situation

▶ Components in teaching critical thinking include

  ▸ Building rapport with each team member

  ▸ Showing how to generate and select a hypothesis

  ▸ Leading students to ask pertinent questions

  ▸ Translating the information into the formulation of problem

  ▸ Demonstrating problem-solving strategies

  ▸ Developing a differential diagnosis, as the final synthesis of the process

▶ Vacek (2009) identified using conceptual approaches with a problem-focused concept map to promote critical thinking and enhancing learning.

▶ Critical thinking skills consist of

  ▹ Analysis

    ▹ Distinguishes the pros and cons, reasons, opinions, and arguments

    ▹ Explores data for relationships

    ▹ Looks for alternative decisions

    ▹ Determines facts from opinions

  ▹ Interpretation

    ▹ Recognizes the client's problems and strengths through verbal, nonverbal, and written data cues

  ▹ Inferences

    ▹ Determines the conclusions based on the data and information available

  ▹ Explanation

    ▹ Justifies reasoning and conclusion in terms of the evidence

    ▹ Constructs a graphic representation of relationship

    ▹ Describes reasoning process in reaching the decision

  ▹ Self-regulation

    ▹ Reconsiders interpretation or judgments based on further information.

    ▹ Examines self for any bias or self-interest (Cise, Wilson, & Thie, 2004)

▶ Concept mapping (see Figure 4–1) can enhance reasoning ability and improve critical thinking skills. It graphically depicts a patient situation to identify correlations among diagnosis, data, pathophysiology, medical orders, procedure results, and collaborative interventions to achieve the patient's goals.

  ▹ Enables providers to see the relationship between what they are thinking and how it relates to the big picture

  ▹ Can be utilized with

    ▹ New graduate residency programs

    ▹ Critical pathways such as core measures

    ▹ Case studies during staff meetings, interdisciplinary patient care rounds, and continuing education programs

FIGURE 4-1.
EXAMPLE OF A CONCEPT MAP EXPLAINING CRITICAL THINKING INTERVENTIONS

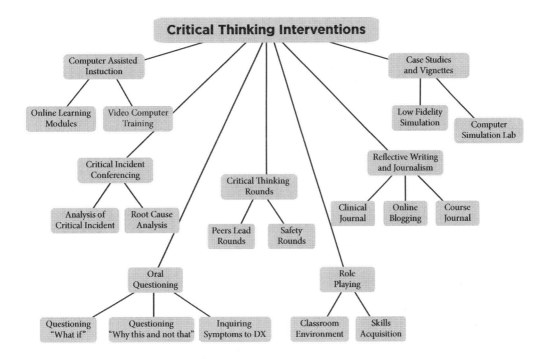

▶ Other effective critical thinking interventions include

   ▹ Reflective writing and journaling

   ▹ Case studies and vignettes

   ▹ Role-playing

   ▹ Critical thinking rounds

   ▹ Critical incident conferencing

   ▹ Oral questioning by clinical faculty and preceptors

   ▹ Computer-assisted instruction

   ▹ Simulations

CLINICAL DECISION-MAKING

▶ Clinical decision-making is a continuous process that includes critical thinking.

▶ The process leads to actions that improve patient care and outcomes and includes

  ▸ Clinical judgment; decision to act considers knowledge of the patient, the patient's normal response, and comparing the current response to the normal response

▶ Clinical reasoning; process of selecting the actions to take. A preceptor can facilitate the process of clinical decision-making by asking questions.

▶ The process steps are:

  ▸ Gather information

  ▸ Generate several hypotheses

  ▸ Narrow down hypotheses and confirm one

  ▸ Implement interventions

  ▸ Evaluate outcomes (Wahl, 2013)

REFERENCES

American Nurses Association and National Nursing Staff Development Organization (2010). *Nursing professional development: Scope and standards of practice.* Silver Spring, MD: Nursesbooks.org.

Armstrong, P. (2009). *Bloom's taxonomy.* Retrieved from http://www.vanderbilt.edu/cft/resources/teaching_resources/theory/blooms.htm

Bastable, S. B., & Doody, J. A. (2008). Behavioral objectives. In S. B. Bastable (Ed.), *Nurse as educator: Principles of teaching and learning for nursing practice* (3rd ed., pp. 383–427). Boston: Jones & Bartlett.

Cise, J., Wilson, C., & Thie, M. (2004). A qualitative tool for critical thinking skill development. *Nurse Educator, 29*(4) 147–151.

Clark, D. (2009). *Bloom's taxonomy of learning domains: The three types of learning.* Retrieved from http://www.nwlink.com/~donclark/hrd/bloom.html

Hardigan, P. C., Cohen, S. R., & Hagen, K. P. (2006). *Bloom's taxonomy.* Retrieved from www.nova.edu/hpdtesting/ctl/forms/bloomstaxonomy.pdf

Huitt, W. (2003). The psychomotor domain. *Educational Psychology Interactive.* Valdosta, GA: Valdosta State University. Retrieved from http://www.edpsycinteractive.org/topics/behavior/psymtr.html

Kelly-Thomas, K. J. (1998). *Clinical and nursing staff development: Current competence, future focus* (2nd ed.). Philadelphia: Lippincott.

Luckowski, A. (2003). Concept mapping as a critical thinking tool for nurse educators. *Journal for Nurses in Staff Development, 19*(5), 225–230.

McManus, N. S. (2009). Domains of learning. In S. L. Bruce (Ed.), *Core curriculum for staff development* (3rd ed., pp. 67–85). Pensacola, FL: National Nursing Staff Development Organization.

McManus, N. S., Maloney, P. L. (2013). Domains of learning. In S. L. Bruce (Ed.), *Core curriculum for nursing professional development* (4th ed., pp. 119–148). Chicago: Association for Nursing Professional Development.

Overbaugh, R. C., & Schultz, L. (2010). *Bloom's taxonomy.* Retrieved from http://ww2.odu.edu/educ/roverbau/Bloom/blooms_taxonomy.htm

Penn, B. K. (2008). How adults learn. In B. K. Penn (Ed.), *Mastering the teaching role: A guide for nurse educators* (pp. 3–18). Philadelphia: F. A. Davis.

Scheckel, M. (2009). Selecting learning experiences to achieve curriculum outcomes. In D. M. Billings & J. A. Halstead (Eds.), *Teaching in nursing: A guide for faculty* (3rd ed., pp. 154–172). St. Louis, MO: Saunders.

Vacek, J. (2009). Using a conceptual approach with concept mapping to promote critical thinking. *Journal of Nursing Education, 45*(6), 212–219.

Wahl, S. E. (2013). Critical thinking and clinical decision making. In S. L. Bruce (Ed.), *Core curriculum for nursing professional development* (4th ed., pp. 291–316). Chicago: Association for Nursing Professional Development.

Walsh, C. M., & Seldomridge, L. A. (2006). Critical thinking: Back to square two. *Journal of Nursing Education, 45*(6), 212–219.

CHAPTER 5

ETHICAL AND LEGAL ISSUES

BACKGROUND

▶ Ethics is an area of study that examines values, actions, and choices to determine right and wrong. Laws are rules of conduct that are enforced by authority. Ethics and law often overlap (American Nurses Association [ANA], 2001; Springhouse, 2009).

▶ A code of ethics makes explicit the values, behaviors, and beliefs that govern appropriate behavior for members of a profession.

▶ According to the *Nursing Professional Development: Scope and Standards of Practice*, "the nursing professional development specialist integrates ethics in all areas of practice" (ANA & National Nursing Staff Development Organization [NNSDO], 2010, p. 37).

▶ The practice of nursing professional development includes ethical responsibilities to self, colleagues, and learners (Condon, 2008).

▶ The nursing professional development specialist provides educational activities on current and emerging ethical topics, including patients' rights, autonomy, end-of-life issues, and confidentiality.

▶ Resources with information about ethical principles and standards that are relevant to nursing professional development include

  » *Nursing Professional Development: Scope and Standards of Practice* (ANA & NNSDO, 2010) identifies 12 criteria that measure how decisions and actions are based on ethical principles.

  » ANA's *Code of Ethics for Nurses with Interpretive Statements* (2001) describes nine provisions of the ethical obligations and duties of every nursing professional.

» ANA's *Guide to the Code of Ethics for Nurses: Interpretation and Application* (2008) provides background information and case examples for each of the ANA code provisions.

» In addition, accrediting organization standards (e.g., The Joint Commission, American Nurses Credentialing Center) and specialty association standards (e.g., Association for Nursing Professional Development) identify ethical standards for nursing practice (ANA, 2010; Chaikin, 2013).

▶ Nursing professional development specialists adhere to all federal, state, and local laws and regulations as well as business and management policies and procedures (American Nurses Credentialing Center [ANCC], 2013b).

▶ Nursing professional development specialists practice in a manner that adheres to ethical principles and respects the codes of ethics of other professionals (ANA & NNSDO, 2010).

ETHICAL ACCOUNTABILITY

▶ Ethical principles include

» *Autonomy:* The right of a competent individual to self-govern or to exercise self-determination

» *Veracity:* Telling the truth

» *Confidentiality:* Protection of personal information

» *Nonmaleficence:* Avoiding harm to and for one's client, specifically the learner in the educational setting

» *Beneficence:* Doing good to and for one's client, the learner

» *Justice:* Fair distribution of resources to all members of society (Nelson, 2008).

▶ Ethical principles are woven throughout the ANA *Code of Ethics for Nurses* (2001) and other key documents that guide the practice of nursing professional development.

▶ The nine provisions of the ANA *Code of Ethics for Nurses* state that the nurse will:

1. Practice with compassion and respect

2. Advocate for and be committed to the patient

3. Promote the health, safety, and rights of the patient

4. Maintain accountability for individual practice and appropriate delegation

5. Preserve integrity and safety

6. Improve healthcare environments and conditions of employment

7. Participate in advancement of the profession

8. Collaborate with others to meet health needs

9. Articulate nursing values and shape social policy (ANA, 2001).

▶ The nursing professional development specialist is responsible for adhering to ethical principles in the assessment, planning, implementation, and evaluation of educational activities and in teacher–learner relationships (ANA & NNSDO, 2010).

▶ The nursing professional development specialist fulfills the following functions related to ethical issues:

  ▸ Offer educational activities on ethical issues and the ethical decision-making process

  ▸ Support staff with knowledge and skills to address situations when patient's wishes are not being honored

  ▸ Facilitate staff access to the ethics committee and ethics resources

  ▸ Serve on the ethics committee or ethics groups

▶ Ethics education should be provided by a nurse ethicist or a nursing professional development specialist who has a comprehensive background in ethics (Chaikin, 2013). Just as *The Code of Ethics for Nurses* (ANA, 2001) addresses provisions for the nurse with respect to patient care, the same terminology can be applied to the prevention of compliance infractions in education:

  ▸ Advocate

  ▸ Maintain accountability

  ▸ Preserve integrity and safety

  ▸ Participate in advancement of the profession

  ▸ Collaborate with others

  ▸ Articulate nursing values

▶ The nursing professional development specialist confronts ethical dilemmas in planning activities just as direct-care nurses confront them at the bedside; they are just different in nature.

▶ Decision-making traps that need to be avoided and corresponding actions to take can be found in Table 5–1.

TABLE 5-1.
ETHICAL DECISION-MAKING TRAPS AND POTENTIAL ACTIONS

TRAP	ACTION
Premature decision-making	Have all the facts at hand
Overconfidence in own judgment	Assemble a planning team
Failing to follow a systematic plan	Develop a planning framework
Inability to recognize the effect of own personal value system	Employ a system of checks and balances

Adapted from "Achieving collaboration in ethical decision-making: Strategies for nurses in practice" by L. Wocial, 1996, *Dimensions in Critical Care Nursing, 15*(3), 150–158.

▶ Curtin (1995) advocates the use of key questions to consider how decisions will affect patient and families, administration, staff, and colleagues.

» "Will anyone be hurt by this decision? Who? Why?"

» "Can this decision or action pass the 'stink' test? If it smells, rethink your priorities" (Curtin, 1995, p. 100).

▶ Approaching the ethical decision-making process this way emphasizes the importance of an individual's perception of decisions while realizing there may be other view points.

LEGAL ACCOUNTABILITY

▶ In the United States, each state has a nurse practice act, enacted by the state legislature, that defines the legal scope of nursing practice within that state. Each state also has a Board of Nursing that establishes and administers the rules and regulations for nursing practice (Springhouse, 2009).

▶ The nursing professional development specialist practices within the legal scope of nursing as described by state nurse practice acts and state boards of nursing.

▶ The nursing professional development specialist is legally responsible to maintain confidentiality within legal and regulatory boundaries, safeguard learners' rights, and use appropriate standards and guidelines to guide practice (ANA & NNSDO, 2010).

JUST CULTURE

▶ "The American Nurses Association (ANA) supports the Just Culture concept and its use in health care to improve patient safety. The ANA supports the collaboration of state boards of nursing, professional nursing associations, hospital associations, patient safety centers and individual health care organizations in developing regional and state-wide Just Culture initiatives" (ANA, 2010 p. 1).

▶ "Just Culture model recognizes that individual practitioners should not be held accountable for system failings over which they have no control. A Just Culture also recognizes many individual or 'active' errors represent predictable interactions between human operators and the systems in which they work. However, in contrast to a culture that touts 'no blame' as its governing principle, a Just Culture does not tolerate conscious disregard of clear risks to patients or gross misconduct (e.g., falsifying a record, performing professional duties while intoxicated)" (ANA, 2010, pp. 2–3).

▶ The Just Culture model describes three types of human behavior that predictably contribute to the occurrence of errors.

    1. Simple human error: Inadvertently doing other than what should have been done

    2. Making a behavioral choice that increases risk where risk is not recognized or is mistakenly believed to be justified

    3. Reckless behavior with conscious disregard for a significant and unjustifiable risk (ANA, 2010)

▶ "The ANA encourages all healthcare organizations to implement a zero tolerance policy related to disruptive behavior, including a professional code of conduct and educational and behavioral interventions to assist nurses in addressing disruptive behavior" (ANA, 2010, p. 7).

▶ The nursing professional development specialist may be involved in educational initiatives to address at-risk behaviors and promote patient safety.

BOUNDARY ISSUES

Conflict of Interest

▶ The potential for conflict of interest exists when "an individual has the ability to control or influence the content of an educational activity **and** has a financial relationship with a commercial interest, the products or services of which are pertinent to the content of the educational activity" (ANCC, 2013b).

▶ The nursing professional development specialist has a responsibility to develop educational activities in a fair and unbiased manner.

▶ The nursing professional development specialist must disclose the presence or absence of any potentially biasing relationship that may be perceived as a conflict of interest. A real or perceived conflict of interest must be identified early in the educational planning process and the specialist must take action to resolve the conflict prior to the implementation of the educational activity.

Commercial Bias

▶ The nursing professional development specialist must be aware of the influence of corporate compliance standards to deter commercial bias in program development.

▶ Commercial bias is an ethical issue indirectly related to fraud and abuse, professional standards, and often conflicts of interest.

▶ The nursing professional development specialist needs to be aware of the ways in which commercial bias may appear and how it may affect the planning of educational activities.

▶ Commercial bias in nursing education is the tendency to make program decisions for presentation that include a narrow view of a topic or situation with the underlying intent and focus on what will attract a larger audience, maximize profit; or showcase a product, process, or person.

▶ Commercial bias is, at times, an outcome of human nature, to make decisions based on intuitive or other cognitive factors rather than evidence-based facts. When the process is not thoroughly thought out, other influences affect decision-making for education planning.

▶ Commercial biases are not only a common outcome of the human thought process during planning; they also drastically skew the reliability of anecdotal, data-based, and legal evidence.

▶ The nursing professional development specialist has a responsibility to develop educational programs free of commercial bias (ANA & NNSDO, 2010).

▶ Develop an action plan to address potential commercial bias in educational activities:

  ▹ Establish a planning committee.

  ▹ Determine acceptable level of bias—10%, 20%? The goal may be 100% bias-free, although the human factor means its attainment is rare.

  ▹ Prepare program evaluation to include questions to solicit participant input on the perception of bias—Yes or No.

  ▹ Consider an additional question—If yes, what contributed to the perception of bias?

  ▹ Review evaluation forms.

  ▹ Follow up with participants when appropriate.

  ▹ In future program development, have an external expert (external to the committee member list) review (Lichti, 2007).

▶ Examples of commercial bias in educational activities:

　▷ Funding by companies not listed as an undesignated educational grant

　▷ Commercial literature distributed within the context of the activity

　▷ Focus on a single product when others are available—an unbalanced presentation

　▷ Recommendations for treatment or practice that are not evidence-based

　▷ Logos and other branding items in presentations

　▷ Trade vs. generic names included unless all products, companies, and trade names are used

Intellectual Property

▶ Intellectual property refers to the ownership and proprietary rights that a person or entity has for creations in the areas of copyrights, trademarks and servicemarks, patents, and trade secrets.

▶ The nursing professional development (NPD) specialist must deal appropriately with ethical dilemmas that arise related to intellectual property ownership. For example, if an NPD specialist creates a learning module in the course of employment, the intellectual property rights to the learning module belong to the employer. Therefore, the NPD specialist may not give or sell the learning module to any person or entity outside the organization (Burrell, 2009).

Plagiarism

▶ Plagiarism is the intentional or unintentional failure to give credit for an idea, statement, etc., that is not one's own (Chaikin, 2013).

▶ Plagiarism through inadequate citation of references or use of another's work without proper credit is a serious concern in educational activities.

▶ Strategies that may be used to avoid plagiarism:

　▷ Use quotation marks to denote the exact wording of statements that come directly from a reference.

　▷ When paraphrasing from a reference, use your own words rather than rearranging or replacing a few words.

　▷ Be meticulous about citing references used in writing (Indiana University, 2004).

▶ If uncertain as to whether information requires a citation, it is better to be cautious and cite rather than risk accusations of plagiarism (Empire State College, 2010; Indiana University, 2004).

Copyright Law

▶ *Copyright* protects the original works of authorship in any tangible medium of expression, such as books, journal articles, sound or video recordings, music, art, plays, movies, computer software, and architecture (U.S. Copyright Office, 2009a).

▶ Copyright does not protect

  ▸ Works that have not been fixed in a tangible form of expression, such as impromptu speeches or performances

  ▸ Titles, names, phrases, symbols, and slogans (although these may be protected as trademarks or servicemarks)

  ▸ Ideas, procedures, processes, concepts, principles

  ▸ Works consisting of information that is common property, such as calendars, height and weight charts, and rulers (U.S. Copyright Office, 2008).

▶ Copyright occurs automatically when a work is created and fixed in a tangible form perceptible to others, such as a book, movie, or musical score.

▶ It is not necessary to register a work with the U.S. Copyright Office for the work to be protected, but registration is necessary to bring a lawsuit for infringement of an American work. Registration is also recommended to document copyright facts for public record and have a certificate as tangible record of registration.

▶ The copyright owner has exclusive rights to do and to authorize any of the following: reproduction or performance of copyrighted work, preparation of derivative works, or distribution of copies.

▶ The use of a copyright notice is not required for new works but may be beneficial because it informs the public that the work is protected by copyright, identifies the copyright owner, and shows the year of initial publication. The letter C within a circle (©), the word "Copyright," or the abbreviation "Copr" indicates copyright.

▶ It is not an infringement of copyright for a library, or any of its employees within the scope of their employment, to reproduce one copy of a work or to distribute a copy, if notice of copyright is included. If a hospital has a subscription to full text access, the subscription covers all employees. The fair use of a copyrighted work for purposes such as criticism, comment, news reporting, scholarship, or research, is not an infringement of copyright. In determining whether use in a specific situation constitutes fair use, four factors must be considered collectively:

  1. Purpose and character of the use, including whether such use is of a commercial nature or is for nonprofit educational purposes

  2. Nature of the copyrighted material (e.g., fiction vs. nonfiction, published vs. unpublished)

3. Amount and substantiality of the portion used in relation to the entire body of work (e.g., fair use for teaching is limited to copying of excerpts up to 1,000 words or 10% of a prose work, or the complete work, if less than 2,500 words; U.S. Copyright Office, 2009b)

4. Effect of the use upon the potential market for or value of the work (U.S. Copyright Office, 2009a).

▸ Copyright issues of special interest to the nursing professional development specialist relate to the use of materials in educational activities. Copyright law applies to the use of any original works of authorship including cartoons, charts, diagrams, graphics, photographs, and videos. Tangible use of any of these in presentations or handouts may violate copyright law unless written copyright permission is obtained. Citing the reference does not forego the need for permission (Burrell, 2009; O'Shea & Robinson, 2002; Turner, 2002; U.S. Copyright Office, 2009a).

▸ If uncertain as to whether use of intellectual property violates copyright, it is better to be cautious and obtain permission for use.

Cheating

▸ Other forms of educational dishonesty that the nursing professional development specialist might encounter in practice include requests to falsify educational records (e.g., competency validation forms) or observation of cheating on a test. While these situations are difficult to address, the specialist must adhere to both legal and ethical standards when they occur (ANA & NNSDO, 2010; Condon, 2008; Johnson, 2009; O'Shea & Robinson, 2002; Turner, 2002).

Confidentiality

▸ *Confidentiality* refers to the protection of information from or about a person.

▸ The nursing professional development specialist establishes and maintains confidentiality of learner and patient information through the use of educational principles, standards, and methodologies (ANA & NNSDO, 2010).

▸ The specialist evaluates factors related to "confidentiality in the use and handling of data, information, and knowledge related to educational programs" (ANA & NNSDO, 2010, p. 37).

▸ The NPD specialist may have access to personal information about learners as well as information from sources such as competency assessments, written exams, and progress evaluations. The specialist should follow established policies and guidelines to protect the privacy and confidentiality of learner information (Johnson, 2009).

REGULATORY CONSIDERATIONS

▶ The American with Disabilities Act (ADA) protects the rights of people with disabilities in the areas of employment and education (Frank, 2009).

▶ The ADA guarantees access to educational opportunities for people with physical and psychological disabilities, including learning disabilities (O'Shea & Robinson, 2002).

▶ The nursing professional development specialist is responsible for making "reasonable accommodations" for learners to fully participate in educational activities (Gunby, 2008).

▶ The Occupational Safety and Health Administration (OSHA) is a division within the U.S. Department of Labor that exists to ensure safe and healthful conditions in the work environment by setting and enforcing standards and by providing training, outreach, education, and assistance. (OSHA, n.d.).

▶ OSHA regulations require healthcare employers to provide education on various topics related to health and safety, including H1N1 virus, bloodborne pathogens, and universal precautions (Ellis & Hartley, 2008).

▶ The nursing professional development specialist is involved in planning, implementing, and evaluating educational activities to meet OSHA mandates.

▶ Pharmaceutical Research and Manufacturers of America (PhRMA) is an organization that represents pharmaceutical research and biotechnology companies. PhRMA works closely with the Food and Drug Administration (FDA) and supports the adverse drug event reporting process.

▶ In addition, PhRMA developed a *Code on Interactions With Healthcare Professionals* in collaboration with the Accreditation Council for Continuing Medical Education (ACCME). This code provided the basis for the standards for disclosure and commercial support in continuing nursing education activities (ANCC, 2013c; PhRMA, 2009).

▶ The ANCC's *Content Integrity Standards for Industry Support in Continuing Nursing Educational Activities* is a resource for the nursing professional development specialist to plan, implement, and evaluate quality continuing nursing education activities with integrity, free from the undue influence of commercial interest organizations (ANCC, 2013c).

▶ The Family Educational Rights and Privacy Act (FERPA) is a federal law that addresses the privacy of student educational records (U.S. Department of Education, 2010).

▶ The nursing professional development specialist must be familiar with FERPA regulations that allow students age 18 and older access to educational records. The law also requires written permission from the eligible student to release information from a student's records except in specific, designated situations.

▶ The Clinical Laboratory Improvement Amendments (CLIA) program is administered by the Centers for Medicare & Medicaid Services to ensure quality laboratory testing on humans.

▶ The nursing professional development specialist must be familiar with educational and competency requirements related to waived testing in clinical settings that were established by CLIA (Centers for Medicare & Medicaid Services, 2010).

PROFESSIONAL STANDARDS

▶ *Professional standards* are statements, often developed by professional organizations, that reflect the values of a profession and describe behavioral expectations for people who practice in that profession (Ellis & Hartley, 2008).

▶ The ANA and NNSDO *Nursing Professional Development: Scope and Standards of Practice* (2010) describes the philosophy, framework, and roles of nursing professional development specialists. The *Scope and Standards* also delineates six standards of practice and 10 standards of professional performance that define expected behaviors for an NPD specialist.

▶ ANCC, a separately incorporated subsidiary of ANA, provides credentialing programs for individuals and organizations in nursing. ANCC offers a certification program to recognize individual nurses in specialty practice areas, an accreditation program to accredit providers and approvers of continuing nursing education, and recognition programs to recognize healthcare organizations for promoting safe, positive work environments (ANCC, 2010).

▶ *Certification* is a voluntary "process by which a nongovernmental agency or an association grants recognition to an individual who has met certain predetermined qualifications" (ANCC, 2013a, p. 4).

▶ *Accreditation* is "a voluntary process by which a nongovernmental agency or organization appraises and grants accredited status to institutions and/or programs or services that meet predetermined structure, process, and outcome criteria" (ANCC, 2013b, p. 3).

▶ ANCC's Commission on Accreditation is responsible for developing and administering the criteria and procedures that govern the process for accreditation of continuing nursing education.

▶ *Continuing nursing education* is defined as a set of learning experiences to build upon the educational and experiential bases of the professional RN to enhance practice, education, administration, research, or theory development and ultimately improve the health of the public and the pursuit of professional career goals (ANCC, 2013b).

▶ An ANCC *accredited provider* is an organization or work unit within an organization that has undergone "an in-depth analysis to determine its capacity to provide quality continuing education" (ANCC, 2013b, p. 4).

▶ An ANCC *accredited approver* is an organization that has undergone an in-depth analysis to determine its capacity to assess and monitor other organizations' compliance with ANCC criteria for quality continuing education, or approve educational activities offered by other organizations or individuals. Accredited approvers fall into one of three categories: constituent and state nurses associations of ANA, specialty nursing organizations, or federal nursing services. Approver units may not approve their own organization's educational activities (ANCC, 2013b).

▶ The term *approved provider* is used to designate an organization or work unit within an organization that has been approved by an accredited approver to provide continuing nursing education activities.

▶ An approved provider and an accredited provider *cannot* approve continuing nursing education activities provided by another organization or institution (ANCC, 2013b).

REFERENCES

American Nurses Association. (2001). *Code of ethics for nurses with interpretive statements.* Washington, DC: American Nurses Publishing.

American Nurses Association. (2008). *Guide to the code of ethics for nurses: Interpretation and application.* Silver Spring, MD: Nursesbooks.org.

American Nurses Association. (2010). *ANA Position Statement; Just culture.* Retrieved from http://www.nursingworld.org/MainMenuCategories/Policy-Advocacy/Positions-and-Resolutions/ANAPositionStatements/Position-Statements-Alphabetically/Just-Culture.html

American Nurses Association & National Nursing Staff Development Organization. (2010). *Nursing professional development: Scope and standards of practice.* Silver Spring, MD: Nursesbooks.org.

American Nurses Credentialing Center. (2010). *About ANCC.* Retrieved from http://www.nursecredentialing.org/FunctionalCategory/AboutANCC.aspx

American Nurses Credentialing Center. (2013a). *Certification general testing and renewal handbook.* Retrieved from http://www.nursecredentialing.org/GeneralTestingRenewalHandbook

American Nurses Credentialing Center. (2013b). *2013 ANCC primary accreditation application manual for providers and approvers.* Silver Spring, MD: Author.

American Nurses Credentialing Center. (2013c). *Content integrity standards for industry support in continuing nursing educational activities.* Retrieved from http://www.nursecredentialing.org/Accreditation/ResourcesServices/Accreditation-CEContentIntegrity

Burrell, T. S. (2009). Ethical and legal principles. In S. L. Bruce (Ed.), *Core curriculum for staff development* (3rd ed., pp. 87–110). Pensacola, FL: National Nursing Staff Development Organization.

Centers for Medicare & Medicaid Services. (2010). *Clinical laboratory improvement amendments overview.* Retrieved from http://www.cms.gov/clia

Chaikin, J. (2013). Ethical and legal principles. In S. L. Bruce (Ed.), *Core curriculum for nursing professional development* (4th ed., pp. 615–640). Chicago: Association for Nursing Professional Development.

Condon, E. H. (2008). Ethical issues in teaching nursing. In B. K. Penn (Ed.), *Mastering the teaching role: A guide for nurse educators* (pp. 401–410). Philadelphia: F. A. Davis.

Curtin, L. (1995). Ethics in management: Creating an ethical organization. *Nursing Management, 26*(9), 96–101.

Dearmon, V. (2009). Risk management and legal issues. In L. Rousell & R. C. Swansburg (Eds.), *Management and leadership for nurse administrators* (5th ed., pp. 470–493). Sudbury, MA: Jones & Bartlett.

Ellis, J. R., & Hartley, C. L. (2008). *Nursing in today's world* (9th ed.). Philadelphia: Lippincott Williams & Wilkins.

Empire State College. (2010). *Library research blog: What is plagiarism and how to avoid it?* Retrieved from http://esclibrary.blogspot.com/2010/04/what-is-plagiarism-and-how-to-avoid-it.html

Frank, B. (2009). Teaching students with disabilities. In D. M. Billings & J. A. Halstead (Eds.), *Teaching in nursing: A guide for faculty* (3rd ed., pp. 53–72). St. Louis, MO: Saunders.

Guido, G. W. (2006). *Legal and ethical issues in nursing* (4th ed.). Upper Saddle River, NJ: Pearson Prentice Hall.

Gunby, S. S. (2008). Legal issues in teaching nursing. In B. K. Penn (Ed.), *Mastering the teaching role: A guide for nurse educators* (pp. 411–420). Philadelphia: F. A. Davis.

Indiana University. (2004). *Plagiarism: What it is and how to recognize and avoid it*. Retrieved from http://www.indiana.edu/~wts/pamphlets/plagiarism.shtml

Johnson, E. G. (2009). The academic performance of students. In D. M. Billings & J. A. Halstead (Eds.), *Teaching in nursing: A guide for faculty* (3rd ed., pp. 33–52). St. Louis, MO: Saunders.

Lichti, A. C. (2007). *CME in practice: Evaluating commercial bias*. Retrieved from http://meetingsnet.com/medical-meetings/cme-practice-evaluating-commercial-bias

Nelson, M. J. (2008). Ethical, legal, and economic foundations of the educational process. In S. B. Bastable (Ed.), *Nurse as educator: Principles of teaching and learning for nursing practice* (3rd ed., pp. 25–49). Boston: Jones & Bartlett.

Occupational Safety & Health Administration. (n.d.). *About OSHA*. Retrieved from http://osha.gov/about.html

O'Shea, K. L., & Robinson, C. B. (2002). Legal and ethical issues in education. In K. L. O'Shea (Ed.), *Staff development nursing secrets* (pp. 59–63). Philadelphia: Hanley & Belfus.

Pharmaceutical Research and Manufacturers of America. (2009). *Code on interactions with healthcare professionals*. Retrieved from http://www.phrma.org/files/2008%2520Profile.pdf

Springhouse. (2009). *Evidence-based nursing guide to legal & professional issues*. Philadelphia: Lippincott Williams & Wilkins.

Tomey, A. M. (2009). *Guide to nursing management and leadership* (8th ed.). St. Louis, MO: Mosby.

Turner, M. (2002). Legal and ethical concerns. In B. E. Puetz & J. W. Aucoin (Eds.), *Conversations in nursing professional development* (pp. 343–347). Pensacola, FL: Pohl Publishing.

U.S. Copyright Office. (2008). *Copyright basics*. Retrieved from http://www.copyright.gov/circs/circ1.pdf

U.S. Copyright Office. (2009a). *Copyright law of the United States and related laws contained in Title 17 of the United States Code.* Retrieved from http://www.copyright.gov/title17/circ92.pdf

U.S. Copyright Office. (2009b). *Reproduction of copyrighted works by educators and librarians.* Retrieved from http://www.copyright.gov/circs/circ21.pdf

U.S. Department of Education. (2010). *Family educational rights and privacy act (FERPA).* Retrieved from http://www2.ed.gov/policy/gen/guid/fpco/ferpa/index.html

Wocial, L. D. (1996). Achieving collaboration in ethical decision-making: Strategies for nurses in practice. *Dimensions in Critical Care Nursing, 15*(3), 150–158.

CHAPTER 6

ISSUES AND TRENDS

PROFESSIONAL ROLE COMPETENCE

▶ According to the American Nurses Association (ANA, 2008), *professional role competence* is performance that meets defined criteria based on the specialty area, context, and model of practice in which an individual nurse is engaged.

▶ Competence begins with academic preparation, licensure, and initial competencies to perform one's job function. Ongoing competence reflects the new, changing, high-risk, and problematic aspects of the job role (Wright, 2005).

ACADEMIC QUALIFICATIONS

▶ Nursing professional development (NPD) specialists should have a graduate degree in nursing or a related discipline from an accredited organization.

▶ If the graduate degree is in a related discipline (e.g., adult education), the baccalaureate degree must be in nursing.

▶ The graduate degree itself is determined by the role of the nursing professional development specialist.

　▷ If the NPD specialist's primary role is specialty or unit-based and she or he functions as both a patient care provider and an educator (e.g., clinical nurse specialist), it may be most appropriate to obtain a graduate degree in nursing with specialty emphasis.

　▷ If the role is primarily that of educator with a focus on program development and implementation, it may be most appropriate to obtain a graduate degree in adult education.

▶ Nursing professional development specialists must demonstrate knowledge of essential education content; the most effective teaching and learning delivery methods; and the skills to plan, develop, implement, and evaluate learning activities.

▶ Persons who function as administrators of nursing professional development departments should optimally possess a doctoral degree in nursing or education. One of the degrees of a nursing professional development administrator must be in nursing (i.e., baccalaureate, master's degree, doctorate).

▶ Administrators must demonstrate not only knowledge of the education process but possess skills in management and business administration (ANA & National Nursing Staff Development Organization [NNSDO], 2010; Avillion, 2005).

LICENSURE

▶ Licensure is a mandatory process by a governmental agency to permit a person to engage in a profession or occupation.

▶ Nursing practice is legally regulated by the definition of nursing in state nurse practice acts.

▶ Legal boundaries are based on interpretation of the safe practice of nursing according to these acts.

▶ State boards of nursing use nursing practice guidelines to issue licenses and protect the welfare of the public.

▶ Nursing professional development specialists are nurses who must be licensed and must practice according to the mandates and guidelines of their nurse practice acts (ANA & NNSDO, 2010).

▶ The nursing professional development specialist must be familiar with the state practice acts and other rules and regulations that apply to the roles he or she teaches.

Nursing Professional Development: Scope and Standards of Practice

▶ The *Scope and Standards* (ANA & NNSDO, 2010) establish the foundational competencies for the nursing professional development specialist.

▶ The ANA first published standards pertaining to this specialty in 1974 as *Standards for Continuing Education in Nursing*.

▶ Revisions were published as *Standards for Nursing Staff Development* in 1990, *Standards for Nursing Professional Development: Continuing Education and Staff Development* in 1994, and *Scope and Standards of Practice for Nursing Professional Development* in 2000.

▶ The *Scope and Standards* support the maintenance of high standards in the delivery of educational programs by describing how the nursing professional development specialist meets the evolving expectations, requirements, demands, and responsibilities of the role (ANA & NNSDO, 2010, p. 9).

Mandatory Education

▶ Professional nurses are expected to be lifelong learners (ANA & NNSDO, 2010; ANA, 2004).

▶ It is essential that all nurses participate in continuing education activities to achieve and maintain competence.

▶ Many states mandate a specific number of hours of continuing education to maintain licensure.

▶ Nurses who hold specialty certifications must participate in a specific number of hours of continuing education and meet other professional development requirements to obtain recertification (American Nurses Credentialing Center [ANCC], 2013).

Portfolio Components

▶ A portfolio is "a portable mechanism for evaluating competencies that may otherwise be difficult to assess, such as practice-based improvements, use of scientific evidence in practice, professional behavior and creative endeavors" (Byrne, Schroeter, Carter & Mower, 2009, as cited in Setter, 2013, p. 516).

▶ Portfolios can be used for performance evaluation, promotion eligibility, pay increases or bonuses, and placement on a career ladder.

▶ The format of a portfolio can vary depending on institutional or individual requirements. Components may include

  ▹ Professional employment

  ▹ Academic preparation: unofficial transcripts, current coursework, copies of degree diplomas

  ▹ Nonacademic education: conferences, specialized training, continuing education

  ▹ Certification documents

  ▹ Contributions to professional nursing organizations

  ▹ Community leadership activities

  ▹ Professional contributions to institution

  ▹ Research and evidence-based practice

- Publications

- Teaching activities

- Special projects

- Awards, recognitions, and supervisor recommendations (Brunt, 2002; Holecek & Foard, 2009)

Changing Focus on Nursing Education Preparation

▶ Increased need for advanced practice nurses.

▶ Doctorate of Nursing Practice to help integrate research into clinical practice.

▶ Institute of Medicine (2011) Future of Nursing report calls for 80% of RNs to be BSN-prepared by 2020.

▶ Academic-clinical practice partnerships and flexible clinical placement schedules.

▶ Increase RN residency programs to improve transition into practice.

CLINICAL PRACTICE AND EXCELLENCE INITIATIVES

▶ The nursing professional development specialist provides educational activities that support an organization's adoption of policies and procedures related to healthcare industry changes and initiatives.

▶ Committee and task force involvement provides the opportunity for the NPD specialist to participate in the design and roll-out of practice and excellence initiatives.

Healthy Work Environment

▶ A healthy work environment is one that provides safety, empowerment, and professional satisfaction and is free of real and perceived threats to health (ANA, 2014).

▶ A healthy work environment supports excellence in nursing practice and patient care.

▶ Kramer and Schmalenberg (2004) identified eight attributes essential for a healthy work environment:

1. Support for education

2. Clinically competent coworkers

3. Collegial and collaborative interprofessional relationships

4. Autonomous nursing practice

5. Control over nursing practice

6. Supportive nurse managers

7. Perceived adequacy of staffing

8. Culture of concern for the patient

▶ Evidence-based standards that are essential for establishing and sustaining healthy work environments have been developed:

▹ Skilled communication with nurses as proficient in communication skills as in clinical skills

▹ True collaboration

▹ Effective decision-making in policy development, clinical care, and organizational operations

▹ Appropriate staffing that matches patient needs with nurse competencies

▹ Meaningful recognition for the value brought to the work of the organization

▹ Authentic leadership that embraces the imperative of a healthy work environment (American Association of Critical-Care Nurses [AACN], 2005)

▶ New knowledge and rapidly changing technology create the need for nurses to have access to planned educational opportunities that will enhance competency, promote job satisfaction, and increase retention (Shirey & Fisher, 2008).

▶ Education that supports a healthy work environment includes orientation, continuing education, internships, educational courses, and degrees (Kramer & Schmalenberg, 2004).

▶ Nursing professional development specialists play a key role in the provision of education supportive of the standards that create and sustain a healthy work environment.

Complex Patient Populations

▶ Aging populations with comorbidities

▶ Chronic disease management

▶ Checklists to ensure standardized processes in operating room, patient handoff, and hourly rounding

▶ Healthcare delivery via primary medical home model

▶ Focus on improved care coordination by healthcare team

▶ Use of crew resource management tools to improve teamwork and communication

Institute for Healthcare Improvement (IHI)

▶ IHI is an independent, nonprofit organization aimed at leading the improvement of health care throughout the world.

▶ IHI has a number of programs for organizations to participate in or use to improve health care according to the Institute of Medicine's six improvement aims: safety, effectiveness, patient-centeredness, timeliness, efficiency, and equity.

▶ The "Triple Aim" of the IHI is to improve the health of communities, the experience of healthcare customers, and the affordability of care.

▶ Examples of past and present programs include The 5 Million Lives Campaign; Improving Outcomes for High-Risk and Critically Ill Patients, which led to the ventilator and central line bundles, rapid response teams, and glucose control interventions; IHI Perinatal Bundles; and prevention of catheter-associated urinary tract infections (Institute for Healthcare Improvement, n.d.).

Centers for Medicare & Medicaid Services (CMS)

▶ A major reimbursement source for hospitals, CMS began decreased reimbursement for nonadherence to quality performance measures in 2001. Value-based incentive payments to hospitals began in 2013 with a focus on achievement or improvement in clinical and patient experience quality measures (Cooke, 2013).

▶ In 2008, CMS eliminated payment for 10 preventable hospital-acquired conditions:

  ▹ Stage III and IV pressure ulcers

  ▹ Fall or trauma resulting in serious injury

  ▹ Vascular catheter–associated infection

  ▹ Catheter-associated urinary tract infection

  ▹ Foreign object retained after surgery

  ▹ Certain surgical site infections

  ▹ Air embolism

  ▹ Blood incompatibility

  ▹ Certain manifestations of poor blood sugar control

  ▹ Certain deep vein thromboses or pulmonary embolisms

▶ CMS also has "never events;" events that should never occur when a patient is being cared for in a hospital. Examples are wrong surgical site on patient, wrong surgery on patient, infant discharged with wrong person, retention of a foreign object in a patient after surgery or procedure, patient death resulting from a fall while being cared for in a hospital, and death or serious disability related to a medication error.

▶ Nursing care influences preventable hospital-acquired conditions and "never events." The NPD specialist has a role in training staff on facility policies and nursing procedures to prevent these events (Hines & Yu, 2009).

The Joint Commission National Patient Safety Goals

▶ The Joint Commission seeks "to continuously improve health care for the public, in collaboration with other stakeholders, by evaluating health care organizations and inspiring them to excel in providing safe and effective care of the highest quality and value" (The Joint Commission, 2014a).

▶ National Patient Safety Goals (NPSGs) were established in 2002 to help hospitals to address specific patient safety concerns. The Joint Commission continues to focus NPSGs on high-priority topics in patient safety and quality care.

▶ An NPSG may be "retired" so the focus stays on the most critical issues. However, retired NPSGs often become part of the standards by which a facility is evaluated for accreditation.

▶ 2014 NPSG topics for hospitals are patient identification, improved communication, medication safety, alarm safety, infection prevention, prevention of mistakes in surgery, and identification of safety risks in patient populations (The Joint Commission, 2014b).

The ANCC Magnet Recognition Program®

▶ The Magnet Program recognizes healthcare organizations for promoting safe, positive work environments that promote the profession of nursing and quality patient outcomes.

▶ Initial research in 1983 led to the identification of 14 Forces of Magnetism. A statistical review of data from 2005 led to a revised model introduced in 2008. The new model groups the 14 Forces of Magnetism into 5 Model Components:

  1. Transformational Leadership

  2. Structural Empowerment

  3. Exemplary Professional Practice

  4. New Knowledge, Innovation, and Improvements

  5. Empirical Quality Results

▶ Magnet designation is seen as a benchmark of quality care (ANCC, 2008a).

▶ Published outcomes related to Magnet designation include:

  » 14% raw mortality rates and 12% lower failure to rescue rates, healthier work environment, and more RNs with BSN degrees and specialty certification in Magnet than in non-Magnet facilities (McHugh, Kelly, Smith, Wu, Vanak, & Aiken, 2013)

  » Higher retention and lower vacancy rates at Magnet facilities: 3.64% vacancy rates compared to 8.1% to 16% vacancy rates in non-Magnet facilities (ANCC, 2009).

The ANCC Pathway to Excellence® Program

▶ The Pathway to Excellence program is a nursing practice excellence recognition that originated from the Texas Nurses Association's Texas Nurse-Friendly Program.

▶ Organizations show how guidelines, known as The Pathway to Excellence Standards, are integrated into operating policies, procedures, and management practices of the healthcare organization.

▶ Standards include:

  » Control of nursing practice

  » Safety of the work environment

  » Systems exist to address patient-care concerns

  » Nurse orientation

  » Chief nursing officer

  » Professional development

  » Competitive wages

  » Nurse recognition

  » Balanced lifestyle

  » Exemplary interdisciplinary collaboration

  » Leadership accountability

  » Quality initiatives (Swartwout, 2009; Wood, 2009)

The ANCC Nursing Skills Competency Program

▶ "ANCC's Nursing Skills Competency Program addresses concerns regarding competency of the nurse by validating that a skills program meets national design standards" (ANCC, 2008b, p. 4).

▶ The program can be used by hospitals, manufacturers or distributors of commercial healthcare products, universities and schools of nursing, temporary staffing agencies, and state nurses associations.

▶ The accreditation is for an educational program, not an organization.

▶ In addition to following the ANCC educational design criteria in continuing education, validity and reliability requirements and selection criteria for faculty must also be demonstrated.

▶ The Nursing Skills Competency Program is a national performance benchmark so nurses may transfer their competency validation from employer to employer (ANCC, 2008b).

CREDENTIALING

▶ Credentialing, according to The Joint Commission (Joint Commission Resources, 2007, pp. 93–94) is "the process of obtaining, verifying, and assessing the qualifications of a health care practitioner to provide patient care services in or for a health care organization."

▶ An organization specifies the minimum credentials required for each job role within the organization.

▶ Credentials include evidence of education, licensure, training, experience, and certifications (Joint Commission Resources, 2007).

Certification

▶ Certification is a process by which a nongovernmental agency or an association validates an individual's knowledge, skills, and abilities in a defined role and clinical area of practice, based on predetermined standards.

▶ Certification can be voluntary or mandatory.

▶ ANCC certification focuses on the individual nurse who has successfully participated in a validation process to ensure appropriate:

  ▹ Knowledge base

  ▹ Skill level

  ▹ Ability to critically think and function in a specialty practice

▶ Certification is now available in most major specialty areas and fosters lifelong learning and enhanced practice.

▶ Most certification eligibility requirements include three common areas of competence:

  ▸ Baccalaureate degree in nursing (a few generalist specialties do not)

  ▸ Working a minimum of 2,000 to 4,000 hours in a period of 3 to 5 years

  ▸ Continuing education or activities to complete required background in the specialty area

▶ "Certification can be used for entry into practice, validation of competence, recognition of excellence, and/or for regulation" (ANCC, 2013, p. 4).

▶ The certifying organization determines the educational credential for professional certification. For example, a baccalaureate in nursing is required for eligibility to take the certification examination in nursing professional development.

▶ The certifying organization also determines the credential that is used upon attaining certification, for example, RN-BC, CCRN.

▶ The Accreditation Board for Specialty Nursing Certification accredits nursing and associated certification programs. The National Commission for Certifying Agencies accredits certification programs and organizations that assess professional competence in the areas of public health, welfare, and safety.

▶ Examples of organizations that provide certification for nursing specialties are American Association of Critical-Care Nurses' Certification Corporation, American Nurses Credentialing Center, National Certification Corporation, and Oncology Nurses Credentialing Certification Corporation.

▶ Certification is good for a term of 5 years. The renewal process for certification, determined by the certifying organization, typically requires continuing education (ANCC, 2013; Kelly-Thomas, 1998).The American Nurses Credentialing Center offers a certification examination in nursing professional development.

Coordinating Activities That Support Certification

▶ Nursing professional development specialists play an important role in assisting professional nurses in attaining and retaining certification in their area of specialty.

▶ How do nursing professional development specialists become catalysts to the process of preparing nurses for certification testing?

  ▸ Assessment—analysis of the learner

    ▹ Knowledge and skills

    ▹ Interview the potential candidate

    ▹ Assess readiness to learn

▹ Interview the nurse manager

▹ Pretest: Use tests found in review books or online (e.g., ANCC website)

▹ Score pretest

▷ Diagnosis and planning

  ▹ Review pretest outcome to determine areas of strength and limitation

  ▹ Develop a strategic plan to enhance areas of limitation

  ▹ Develop the content

  ▹ Obtain materials from various resources (e.g., ANCC provides test content outlines free on its website)

    ▷ Incorporate a prepared curriculum

    ▷ Individualize to the nurse's needs

    ▷ Prepare to address areas of limitation and reinforce strengths if planning for a group

  ▹ Develop teaching materials

  ▹ Develop timeline for education

    ▷ Gantt chart for visual of expectations and sequence of education

▷ Implementation

  ▹ Initiate strategic plan

  ▹ Encourage study groups

  ▹ Schedule review sessions

  ▹ Vary learning aids

    ▷ Self-learning modules

    ▷ Lecture

    ▷ Incorporate online education, such as

      ← Distance learning programs

      ← Webinars

      ← CNE provider company products

    ▷ ANCC offers review courses in person and online

    ▷ Several nursing organizations offer their own review courses (e.g., Association for Nursing Professional Development [ANPD] for nursing staff development [NPD] certification, AACN for critical care)

- Evaluation

  - Posttest

  - Analyze achievement

  - Compare to pretest and precourse performance

  - Validate progress with manager

  - Validate course success with participants

  - Revise plan as needed

- Champion any of the following, if not currently in place:

  - Organizational recognition for certification

    - Full or partial certification reimbursement

    - Salary increases

    - Certification pay attached to base salary

    - One-time bonus

    - Unit-based plaque with names of certified nurses, including dates of certification, kept current

    - Nursing or organization newsletter recognition

    - Celebration of Certified Nurses Day in March or during Nurses' Day activities

    - Recognition in nursing periodicals

- Encourage nurses to complete their professional continuing education requirements

- Maintain a database of certified nurses with area of specialty, date of certification, and date of upcoming recertification

- Assist nurses to recertify when due; a gentle reminder works well

▶ Certification plays an important part in the advancement of a career and the profession (Yoder-Wise, 2007, p. 572).

Certificates

▶ Certificates are obtained for clinical practice skills based on safety and standards of care. Examples include basic cardiac life support, neonatal resuscitation program, fetal heart-rate monitoring, and chemotherapy administration.

▶ These certificates require a renewal process demonstrating the skill to ensure competency is maintained.

▶ Nursing professional development specialists often have the credentials to be instructors in programs that provide these certifications.

▶ Healthcare institutions also may establish standards by which staff are certified to perform specific skills within that organization such as IV insertion, Foley insertion, and telemetry monitoring.

▶ The nursing professional development specialist provides the training and validation of institution-based certification.

PRACTICE BASED ON EVIDENCE

Background

▶ Evidence-based practice (EBP) is a problem-solving method that integrates

  ▹ The search and critical appraisal of relevant data to answer a clinical question,

  ▹ One's own clinical expertise, and

  ▹ The patient's preferences and values (Melnyk & Fineout-Overholt, 2005).

▶ Research utilization differs from EBP in that research utilization uses knowledge typically based on a single study.

▶ EBP can be applied to the practice of nursing professional development by using data related to the practice of teaching, the educator's expertise, and learner characteristics.

▶ Content for educational programs is to be evidenced-based.

Five Steps of Evidence-Based Practice

▶ Step 1: Formulate the burning clinical question in the PICO format:

  ▹ **Patient population**

  ▹ **Intervention of interest**

  ▹ **Comparison intervention or status**

  ▹ **Outcome**

▶ Step 2: Search for best evidence from a hierarchy of evidence.

▶ Step 3: Conduct a critical review of the evidence.

▶ Step 4: Integrate the evidence with the provider's expertise, assessment of the patient, available resources, and the patient's preferences.

▶ Step 5: Evaluate the effectiveness of the evidenced-based intervention in meeting the desired outcome (Melnyk & Fineout-Overholt, 2005).

Sources of Evidence

▶ *Literature:* Literature is one of the most accessible forms of evidence. Published literature can be limited due to researchers' failure to publish, a reluctance to share proprietary information, and English language journals typically preferring to publishing positive findings (Malloch & Porter-O'Grady, 2006).

▶ *Databases:* Many databases with healthcare information can be accessed free of charge or for a fee from a vendor. Vendor-access subscription is typically done by an organization. While there may be some overlap, each database has a specific focus. The most commonly used databases for clinical content are

   » Cochrane Database of Systematic Reviews: Full text of regularly updated systematic reviews; contains seven different databases (http://www.cochrane.org)

   » National Guideline Clearinghouse: Summaries of guidelines based on scientific evidence or consensus of expert opinion; supported by the Agency for Healthcare Research and Quality (AHRQ; http://www.guideline.gov)

   » PubMed: A catalog of over 4,600 biomedical journals' citations, usually with abstracts (full text articles are available from journal vendors); produced by the National Library of Medicine; organized by medical subject headings as well as searchable by citation (http://www.ncbi.nlm.nih.gov/sites/entrez)

   » Cumulative Index of Nursing and Allied Health Literature (CINAHL): Citations with available abstracts from 13 nursing, allied health, and bioscience areas; includes journals, books, drug monographs, dissertations, and images (http://www.ebscohost.com/cinahl/)

   » PsycINFO: Scholarly literature including books and dissertations in behavioral sciences; available through American Psychological Association (APA) or Ovid (http://www.apa.org/pubs/databases/psycinfo/index.aspx; Melnyk & Fineout-Overholt, 2005)

   » Educational Resources Information Center (ERIC): Bibliographic records of journal articles and other education-related materials (http://www.eric.ed.gov/)

   » Quality and Safety Education for Nurses (QSEN): Funded by the Robert Wood Johnson Foundation, QSEN has annotated bibliographies and teaching strategies essential to the development of quality and safety competencies (http://www.qsen.org/)

▶ *Reliable sources:* Clinical trials are one of the most reliable sources, although results need to be generalizable to the current situation. Source credibility can be based on past accomplishments, publications in peer-reviewed journals, and association with specialty organizations (Malloch & Porter-O'Grady, 2006; Melnyk & Fineout-Overholt, 2005).

▶ *Expert opinion:* Expert opinion can be used as an adjunct to research data, or when there is a lack of or conflict in research-based studies. Expert opinion can be found at conferences, professional websites, or from clinical experts (Malloch & Porter-O'Grady, 2006).

▶ *Best practices:* Best practices are protocols and practices based on standards that have quality clinical and financial outcomes (Malloch & Porter-O'Grady, 2006)

REFERENCES

American Association of Critical-Care Nurses. (2005). AACN *standards for establishing and sustaining healthy work environments.* Aliso Viejo, CA: Author.

American Nurses Association & National Nursing Staff Development Organization. (2010). *Nursing professional development: Scope and standards of practice.* Silver Spring, MD: Nursesbooks.org.

American Nurses Association. (1974). *Standards for continuing education in nursing.* Kansas City, MO: American Nurses Publishing.

American Nurses Association. (1990). *Standards for nursing staff development.* Kansas City, MO: American Nurses Publishing.

American Nurses Association. (1994). *Standards for nursing professional development: Continuing education and staff development.* Washington, DC: American Nurses Publishing.

American Nurses Association. (2000). *Scope and standards of practice for nursing professional development.* Washington, DC: American Nurses Publishing.

American Nurses Association. (2004). *Nursing scope and standards of practice.* Washington, DC: American Nurses Publishing.

American Nurses Association. (2008). *Professional role competence.* Retrieved from http://nursingworld.org/MainMenuCategories/Policy-Advocacy/Positions-and-Resolutions/ANAPositionStatements/Position-Statements-Alphabetically/Professional-Role-Competence.html

American Nurses Association. (2014). *Healthy work environment.* Retrieved from http://www.nursingworld.org/MainMenuCategories/WorkplaceSafety/Healthy-Work-Environment

American Nurses Credentialing Center. (2008a). *A new model for ANCC's Magnet Recognition Program* [Brochure]. Silver Spring, MD: Author.

American Nurses Credentialing Center. (2008b). *Overview of ANCC Nursing Skills Competency Program: A new kind of nursing accreditation* [Brochure]. Silver Spring, MD: Author.

American Nurses Credentialing Center. (2009). *The business case for Magnet: A CNO toolkit.* Silver Spring, MD: Author

American Nurses Credentialing Center. (2013). *2013 certification general testing and renewal handbook.* Silver Spring, MD: Author.

Avillion, A. E. (2005). *Nurse educator manual: Essential skills and guidelines for effective practice.* Marblehead, MA: HCPro.

Brunt, B. A. (2002). Standards of practice. In B. E. Puetz & J. W. Aucoin (Eds.), *Conversations in nursing professional development* (pp. 365–372). Pensacola, FL: Pohl Publishing.

Cooke, M. (2013). Issues and trends in nursing professional development. In S. L. Bruce (Ed.), *Core curriculum for nursing professional development.* (4th ed., pp. 587–613). Chicago: Association for Nursing Professional Development.

Hines, P. A., & Yu, K. M. (2009). The changing reimbursement landscape: Nurses' role in quality and operational excellence. *Nursing Economic$, 27*(1), 7–13.

Holecek, A., & Foard, M. (2009). Promoting a culture of professionalism: The birth of the nursing portfolio. *Nurse Leader, 7*(6), pp. 30–35.

Institute for Healthcare Improvement. (n.d.). *Topics.* Retrieved from http://www.ihi.org/topics/Pages/default.aspx http://www.ihi.org/ihi/programs

Institute of Medicine. (2011). *The future of nursing: Leading change, advancing health.* Washington, DC: National Academies Press.

Joint Commission, The. (2014a). *Facts about The Joint Commission* [Fact Sheet]. Retrieved from http://www.jointcommission.org/about_us/fact_sheets.aspx

Joint Commission, The. (2014b). *2014 National patient safety goals.* Retrieved from http://www.jointcommission.org/assets/1/6/2014_HAP_NPSG_E.pdf

Joint Commission Resources. (2007). *Assessing hospital staff competencies* (2nd ed.). Oakbrook Terrace, IL: Joint Commission on Accreditation of Healthcare Organizations.

Kelly-Thomas, K. J. (1998). *Clinical and nursing staff development: Current competence, future focus* (2nd ed.). Philadelphia: Lippincott.

Kramer, M., & Schmalenberg, C. (2004). Development and evaluation of essentials of magnetism tool. *The Journal of Nursing Administration, 34*(7/8), 365–378.

Malloch, K., & Porter-O'Grady, T. (2006). *Introduction to evidence-based practice in nursing and health care.* Boston: Jones & Bartlett.

McHugh, M., Kelly. L., Smith, H., Wu, E., Vanak, J., & Aiken, L. (2013). Lower mortality in Magnet hospitals. *Medical Care, 51*(5): 382–388.

Melnyk, B. M., & Fineout-Overholt, E. (2005). *Evidence-based practice in nursing & healthcare: A guide to best practice.* Philadelphia: Lippincott Williams & Wilkins.

Setter, R. (2013). Career development and role transition. In S. L. Bruce (Ed.), *Core curriculum for nursing professional development.* (4th ed., pp. 515–525). Chicago: Association for Nursing Professional Development.

Shirey, M. R., & Fisher, M. L. (2008). Leadership agenda for change toward healthy work environments in acute and critical care. *Critical Care Nurse, 28*(5):66–78.

Swartwout, E. (2009). *ANCC Pathway to Excellence.* Silver Spring, MD: American Nurses Credentialing Center. Retrieved from http://www.nursecredentialing.org/Pathway

Wood, D. (2009). *ANCC's Pathway to Excellence: Commitment to good nursing environments.* AMN Healthcare. Retrieved from http://www.nursezone.com/Nursing-News-Events/more-features/ANCC%E2%80%99s-Pathway-to-Excellence-Commitment-to-Good-Nursing-Environments_32216.aspx

Wright, D. (2005). *The ultimate guide to competency assessment in health care* (3rd ed.). Minneapolis, MN: Creative Health Care Management.

Yoder-Wise, P. (2007). *Leading and managing in nursing* (4th ed.). St. Louis, MO: Mosby.

CHAPTER 7

FUNCTIONS OF THE NURSING PROFESSIONAL DEVELOPMENT SPECIALTY

BACKGROUND

▶ "Nursing professional development is a specialized nursing practice that facilitates the professional development of nurses in their participation in lifelong learning activities to enhance their professional competence and role performance" (American Nurses Association [ANA] and National Nursing Staff Development Organization (NNSDO), 2010, p. 3).

▶ In the educator role, nursing professional development specialists provide orientation, inservice, and continuing education.

▶ Orientation includes preceptor development and competency assessment, in addition to learning activities to help new employees learn their roles within the organization.

▶ Inservice entails using different teaching methods to educate staff on how to perform in their roles within the organization.

▶ Continuing education involves educational activities that are designed to enhance knowledge, skills, or attitudes regardless of the participant's employer.

ORIENTATION

▶ Orientation is "the process of introducing nursing staff to the philosophy, goals, policies, procedures, role expectations, and other factors needed to function in a specific work setting" (ANA, 2010, p. 5).

▶ Orientation occurs for employees new to an organization and when an employee changes roles, responsibilities, or practice settings within an organization.

▶ Aspects of orientation include job description; organizational and departmental policies and procedures; information management; performance improvement process; regulatory requirements; patient population-specific considerations; and competency assessment for role-specific duties, documentation, and equipment (Kelly-Thomas, 1998; O'Shea, 2002).

▶ The length of orientation varies according to the knowledge, skills, and abilities required for the position and the experience of the employee.

▶ Role transition requires that the employee learn the values, expected behaviors, and essential knowledge to perform her or his role competently in the organization (O'Shea, 2002).

▶ Developing competence is accomplished through "processes and programs designed to cultivate, generate, and extend the competence of nurses related to expectations and performance standards new to the person or new to the organization" (Kelly-Thomas, 1998, p. 26).

▶ "Competency-based education (CBE) is an alternative approach to instruction that emphasizes a learner's ability to demonstrate integration of the knowledge, attitudes, and skills that are most important to a particular task, activity, or role" (Alspach, 1995).

▶ Learning activities are designed to meet regulatory, organizational, departmental, unit, and role requirements of orientation.

▶ The goals of orientation are clearly defined so all parties involved (orientee, preceptor, educator, supervisor) are clear about their function within and expectations of the orientation process.

▶ The nursing professional development specialist oversees the unit-based orientation process by meeting with the orientee, preceptor, and employee's supervisor to ensure progress is being made toward goals of orientation (Alspach, 1995; Kelly-Thomas, 1998).

PRECEPTOR DEVELOPMENT

▶ A successful orientation occurs in a precepted, role-modeled environment.

▶ The roles of a preceptor include that of educator, role model, and socializer.

   ▻ Educator: Assesses the new hire's learning needs, plans learning activities, implements the teaching plan, and evaluates the orientee's performance.

   ▻ Role model: Demonstrates how the nurse is expected to perform the job.

   ▻ Socializer: Makes the orientee feel welcome and helps her or him to integrate socially and professionally with peer group, unit, and hospital (Alspach, 1995, 2002).

▶ Preceptor characteristics include desire to teach positive interpersonal skills, exceptional clinical performance, leadership, and adherence to organizational policy and procedures.

▶ Collaboratively, the nursing professional development (NPD) specialist and the manager identify employees who exemplify the characteristics needed of preceptors.

▶ Development of a group of employees who understand the preceptor role and its important function within the organization is the responsibility of the nurse educator.

▶ Content to include in a preceptor training program:

   ▻ Principles of adult learning

   ▻ Role of the preceptor

   ▻ Clinical instruction strategies

   ▻ Relationship building

   ▻ Cultural and multigenerational diversity

   ▻ Conflict resolution

   ▻ Performance coaching

   ▻ Feedback and evaluation (Harper & Rooney, 2013, pp. 783–784)

▶ The preceptor requires support before, during, and after each preceptorship experience from the NPD specialist and the nurse manager.

   ▻ Before:

      ▷ NPD specialist: Provide a formal, effective preceptor training program and a written preceptor job description

      ▷ Nurse manager: Provide orientee's resume and self-assessment, interview findings, and compensation in either a financial or career ladder form

▸ During:

▹ NPD specialist: Maintain close contact to guide the teaching-learning process, address questions, troubleshoot problems, and monitor effectiveness and progress of the program

▹ Nurse manager: Align schedule of preceptor and orientee and ensure staffing is adequate to meet teaching-learning needs

▸ After:

▹ NPD specialist: Provide regularly scheduled preceptor support groups and continuing education programs on advanced preceptor topics, such as matching teaching and learning styles or creative clinical teaching strategies

▹ Nurse manager: Provide a means of recognition and reward and time away from precepting to prevent burnout or meet preceptor's personal needs (Alspach, 1995)

COMPETENCY MANAGEMENT

▶ "Competence is a potential and/or capacity to function in a given situation" (American Board of Nursing Specialities, 2011, as cited in Wright, 2013, p. 500).

▶ "Competency is the application of knowledge, skills, and behaviors that are needed to fulfill organizational, departmental, and work setting requirements under varied circumstances of the real world" (Wright, 2005, p. 8).

▶ Competence assessment is a continual process that begins when leaders define the competencies required of a job position and continues with regular validation of a person's attainment and maintenance of these competencies (Joint Commission Resources, 2007).

▶ Competencies are broad statements describing general areas of behavior in a particular role and work setting (Alspach, 1995; Joint Commission Resources, 2007) that should:

▸ Describe a general category of behavior

▸ Be focused on the learner

▸ Be behavioral and measurable

▸ Be free from performance conditions

▸ Be validated by experts (Kelly-Thomas, 1998)

▶ Competency statements are written around an organizing framework based on the organization's preference. Example frameworks include nursing diagnoses, nursing process, therapies, nursing practice standards, and medical diagnoses (Alspach, 1995; Kelly-Thomas, 1998).

▶ The development of competency statements and performance criteria is a collaborative effort among the nurse educator, nurse manager, clinical nurse specialists, and select nursing staff members (Alspach, 1995).

▶ Core or initial competencies focus on the knowledge, skills, and abilities needed to perform the job role in the first 6 to 12 months, are grouped into clusters (e.g., communication, care management), and capture the overall job goals (Kelly-Thomas, 1998; Wright, 2005).

▶ Ongoing competencies reflect the ever-changing nature of the job and the organization's missions and goals (Wright, 2005).

▶ Ongoing competencies focus on new skills, new products, changes in practice or equipment, and skills that are high-risk, low-volume, or problem-prone (Stafford, 2002; Wright, 2005).

▶ Various methods may be used to prioritize identified ongoing competencies because the validation process cannot include all competencies. Time, resources, and meaningfulness are considerations for an efficient and cost-effective ongoing competency assessment process.

   ▹ Alspach's (1995) Four Priority Factors

      1. Fatal: High-risk aspects of patient care needs.

      2. Fundamental: Essential aspects of effective nursing practice.

      3. Frequency: Area of nursing practice that is performed often.

      4. Facility/Fixed: Requirement of external accrediting agency or healthcare organization.

   ▹ Wright (2005)

      ▹ Is the job aspect in more than one category: new, change, high-risk, problematic?

      ▹ Does the outcome of the competency have an outcome for the patient, customer, or employee?

      ▹ Regarding high-risk job aspects, is it time-sensitive (performance does not allow time to "look it up")?

▶ The nursing professional development specialist works collaboratively with management to identify ongoing competencies and methods for measuring competence.

▶ The validation process includes many different methods to recognize individual differences in learning styles, demonstration preferences, and experience levels. Wright (2005) recommends increasing the difficulty or hassle-factor of validation for the learner as time goes on to prevent laggards in the competence assessment process.

▶ Verification methods can include tests and exams, return demonstration, evidence of daily work, case studies, examplars, peer review, self-assessment, discussion and reflection groups, mock events, presentations, and quality improvement monitors (Wright, 2013).

▶ Employees are accountable for ensuring that validation of their competencies occurs; managers are accountable to create systems to support competency assessment (Wright, 2005).

▶ Assessing competence is done through "processes and programs designed to measure and evaluate the competency of nurses in relation to expected performance standards" (Kelly-Thomas, 1998, p. 26).

INSERVICE

▶ Inservices are "learning experiences that help individuals perform within a given job role in a specific setting" (Wilson, 2013, p. 575).

▶ Inservices are a quick response to changes in the work environment (Misko, 2009).

▶ Learner experiences that take place during work hours in the workplace are also referred to as on-the-job or just-in-time training (Avillion, 2005, 2008).

▶ Inservice characteristics:

  ▹ Shorter duration (15 to 60 minutes per session)

  ▹ More informal structure and presentation styles

  ▹ Conducted in or immediately adjacent to the work site

  ▹ Shorter interval between instruction and evaluation of learning

  ▹ May involve faculty who are not hospital staff members

  ▹ Often involve only small group of learners (Alspach, 1995, p. 237)

▶ Inservice education methodology depends on the program objectives and learner needs. Methods may include formal lectures, discussions, poster presentations, self-paced learning techniques, and train-the trainer (Avillion, 2005, 2008).

▶ Content may include commonly referred to "mandatories:" fire safety, back safety, infection control, electrical safety, radiation safety, bloodborne pathogens, and other regulatory, state, and organization requirements.

▶ The manuals of the accrediting bodies delineate training requirements. Often the organization states the specifics of the requirements within its policies (O'Shea, 2002).

▶ The nursing professional development specialist partners with other departments, for example, infection control and risk management, to identify organizational requirements for inservice content.

▶ Inservice education also can be incidental learning based on patient situations, medications, and needs. Other informal learning occurs during patient care rounds, discharge planning rounds, and reflection on clinical practice (Alspach, 1995).

▶ The nursing professional development specialist needs to accommodate the learning needs of staff on all shifts. Methodologies that can be employed are self-learning packets, video with posttests, computer-assisted instruction, designated night and weekend educators, or rotation to nights for educational needs.

▶ Inservices may be provided by vendor representatives; however, the NPD specialist should review the content for appropriateness and ensure it is more than a marketing strategy. Vendor educators can be an excellent source of inservice material and developing collegial relationships with company representatives can be beneficial to the educator and the organization.

▶ Successful inservices depend on the ability of the NPD specialist, availability of equipment, and readiness of the learner. Involve managers to increase attendance at mandatory inservices (Alspach, 1995; Kelly-Thomas, 1998).

CONTINUING EDUCATION

▶ Continuing nursing education activities are "those learning activities intended to build upon the educational and experiential bases of the professional RN for the enhancement of practice, education, administration, research, or theory development to the end of improving the health of the public and RNs' pursuit of their professional career goals" (American Nurses Credentialing Center [ANCC], 2013, p. 102).

▶ Continuing nursing education (CNE) is viewed as an employee benefit, necessary for continued competence, required for advanced certification, and may be needed for licensure.

▶ Some states require a specific number of continuing education hours for relicensure; other states may be more prescriptive and require the education be in a certain area such as restraints or forensic evidence collection.

▶ Some boards of nursing accept CNE activities that have been provided by an ANCC-accredited provider or approved by an ANCC-accredited approver. Others have developed their own mechanisms for approval of CNE activities.

▶ The nursing professional development curriculum is designed to meet the continuing education (CE) needs of the organization's employees to meet organizational goals and contribute to safe health care (Kelly-Thomas, 1998).

▶ Continuing education in one's specialty is often required to maintain national certification (ANCC, 2006).

▶ Continuing education activities fall under the function of a nursing professional development department, but may also be offered by independent agencies, entrepreneurs, or universities (Alspach, 1995).

▶ The American Nurses Credentialing Center (ANCC) Accreditation Program has established criteria to ensure that educational activities are planned, implemented, and evaluated using educational standards and adult learning principles (ANCC, 2013).

▶ The National League of Nursing (NLN) is an Authorized Provider of continuing education by the International Association for Continuing Education and Training. NLN CE programs are limited to those that promote the nursing faculty role (NLN, 2013).

▶ In addition to content, the time and cost required to develop and evaluate a CE offering is important to consider when deciding to offer contact hours for an educational activity.

▶ Continuing nursing education is measured in contact hours calculated from the amount of the educational activity's content that is devoted to transmitting new or transferable knowledge. "A contact hour is 60 minutes of organized learning. Contact hours cannot be rounded up but can be rounded down to 1/10th or 1/100th" (ANCC, 2011, as cited in Green, 2013, p. 210).

▶ CE can be provided in a number of formats:

  ⁕ Workshop: Typically a single day for a small group covering in-depth content; may be skill-based with hands-on opportunities

  ⁕ Seminar: A small group that exchanges information about a specific topic; requires preparation by the learner

  ⁕ Conference: Group process format involving participant discussion related to a single topic area; typically has a coordinator and may last multiple days

  ⁕ Course: Comprehensive study of a topic area through a series of learning activities lasting a few days; different than academic courses

» Institute: Formal learning experiences with experts presenting information to participants; often a multiday program

» Symposium: Two or more experts presenting information on a topic, followed by a moderator summary and then a question-and-answer period; can accommodate larger audiences

» Self-study: Varied formats that can include programmed instruction, self-learning packages, reading books or journals, and computer-assisted instruction including online modules, webinars, podcasts, and so on (Alspach, 1995)

CLINICAL AFFILIATIONS

▶ The nursing professional development specialist may be the coordinator for clinical affiliation placements within the healthcare organization.

▶ Clinical affiliations begin with a memorandum of agreement or contract between the academic institution and the healthcare organization. This contract states the responsibilities of the academic institution, the healthcare organization, the faculty, and the student.

▶ The nursing professional development specialist works with managers of units and areas to identify their willingness and ability to support students within their areas.

▶ Student learning objectives are obtained from the academic institution to ensure they can be met in the specific clinical areas.

▶ The nursing professional development specialist maintains a schedule of dates and times of clinical group assignment to avert double assignment and unit staff burnout.

▶ Methodologies to orient faculty to the organization include attendance at nursing or per-diem (agency) orientation, self-study packets, or computer-assisted instruction, as well as a brief precepted experience on the unit where the faculty member will have students (Duffy, 2001; Stafford, 2009).

▶ Faculty orientation includes competency in point-of-care or waived testing, medication administration, and documentation.

▶ Methodologies to orient students include school group orientation by the NPD specialist, clinical group orientation by faculty, self-study packets, or computer-assisted instruction.

▶ Other clinical affiliation coordinator duties can include oversight of confidentiality policy, processes for obtaining facility access badges and computer system access, and ensuring compliance with regulatory requirements.

▶ Faculty are responsible for supervision and evaluation of clinical nursing student performance; the healthcare institution is responsible for patient care (Duffy, 2001).

REFERENCES

Alspach, J. G. (1995). *The educational process in nursing staff development.* St. Louis, MO: Mosby.

Alspach, J. G. (2002). Preceptor development. In B. E. Puetz & J. W. Aucoin (Eds.) *Conversations in nursing professional development* (pp. 261–272). Pensacola, FL: Pohl Publishing.

American Nurses Association and National Nursing Staff Development Organization. (2010). *Nursing professional development: Scope and standards of practice.* Silver Spring, MD: Nursesbooks.org.

American Nurses Credentialing Center. (2006). *Manual for accreditation as an approver or provider of continuing education: Application manual.* Silver Spring, MD: Author.

American Nurses Credentialing Center. (2013). *2013 ANCC primary accreditation application manual for providers and approvers.* Silver Spring, MD: Author.

Avillion, A. E. (2005). *Nurse educator manual: Essential skills and guidelines for effective practice.* Marblehead, MA: HCPro.

Avillion, A. E. (2008). *A practical guide to staff development: Tools and techniques for effective education* (2nd ed.). Marblehead, MA: HCPro.

Duffy, M. M. (2001). Arranging clinical affiliations. *Journal for Nurses in Staff Development, 17,* 41–43.

Green, D. A. (2013). Educational planning. In S. L. Bruce (Ed.), *Core curriculum for nursing professional development* (4th ed., pp. 197–228). Chicago: Association for Nursing Professional Development.

Harper, M. G., & Rooney, E. (2013). Elements of nursing professional development practice: educator/academic liaison. In S. L. Bruce (Ed.), *Core curriculum for nursing professional development* (4th ed., pp. 779–797). Chicago: Association for Nursing Professional Development.

Joint Commission Resources. (2007). *Assessing hospital staff competence* (2nd ed.). Oakbrook Terrace, IL: Joint Commission on Accreditation of Healthcare Organizations.

Kelly-Thomas, K. J. (1998). *Clinical and nursing staff development: Current competence, future focus* (2nd ed.). Philadelphia: Lippincott.

Misko, L. (2009). Implementation of learning activities. In S. L. Bruce (Ed.) *Core curriculum for staff development* (pp. 251–278). Pensacola, FL: National Nursing Staff Development Organization.

National League of Nursing. (2013). *Continuing education.* Retrieved from http://www.nln.org/ContinuingEd/index.htm

O'Shea, K. L. (2002). *Staff development nursing secrets.* Philadelphia: Hanley & Belfus.

Speers, A. T., Strzyzewski, N., & Ziolkowski, L. D. (2004). Preceptor preparation: An investment in the future. *Journal for Nurses in Staff Development, 20*(3), 127.

Stafford, R. (2002). Nursing staff development. In B. E. Puetz & J. W. Aucoin (Eds.) *Conversations in nursing professional development* (pp. 35–42). Pensacola, FL: Pohl Publishing.

Wilson, C. M. (2013). Professional practice guidelines. In S. L. Bruce (Ed.), *Core curriculum for nursing professional development* (4th ed., pp. 571–585). Chicago: Association for Nursing Professional Development.

Wright, D. (2005). *The ultimate guide to competency assessment in health care.* Minneapolis: Creative Health Care Management.

Wright, D. (2013). Competency programs. In S. L. Bruce (Ed.), *Core curriculum for nursing professional development* (4th ed., pp. 499–513). Chicago: Association for Nursing Professional Development.

CHAPTER 8

EDUCATIONAL PROCESS

BACKGROUND

▶ Nursing professional development is a specialized nursing practice that can be illustrated using a model with inputs, throughputs, outputs, and feedback.

▶ *Nursing Professional Development: Scope and Standards of Practice* (American Nurses Association [ANA] and National Nursing Staff Development Organization [NNSDO], 2010) describes six standards of practice for the nursing professional development specialist related to the educational process.

   ▹ Standard 1. Assessment: "Collects data and information related to educational needs and other pertinent situations" (p. 23)

   ▹ Standard 2. Identification of issues and trends: "Analyzes issues, trends, and supporting data to determine the needs of individuals, organizations, and communities" (p. 24)

   ▹ Standard 3. Outcomes identification: "Identifies desired outcomes" (p. 25)

   ▹ Standard 4. Planning: "Establishes a plan that prescribes strategies, alternatives, and resources to achieve expected outcomes" (p. 26)

   ▹ Standard 5. Implementation: "Implements the identified plan" (p. 27)

   ▹ Standard 6. Evaluation: "Evaluates progress toward attainment of outcomes" (p. 31)

▶ An educational activity is "a planned, organized effort aimed at accomplishing educational objectives" (Green, 2013, p. 220).

▶ An educational activity may be in one or more different forms (e.g., lecture, seminar, conference, independent study, simulation, web-based).

▶ The American Nurses Credentialing Center (ANCC, 2013) has defined criteria for the needs assessment, planning, implementation, and evaluation of continuing nursing education activities that can be applied to any educational activity. These criteria incorporate adult learning principles as well as professional standards and ethics.

SYSTEMS THEORY

▶ Systems theory was developed by Ludwig von Bertalanffy in the 1950s to examine how living organisms processed elements and the effects of internal and external factors.

▶ Systems theory is the interaction between complex elements (Figure 8–1).

   ▸ It looks at the structural elements of an organization in terms of input, throughputs, outputs, and the interrelationships between them.

   ▸ Subsystems help define the internal environments.

   ▸ A suprasystem defines the external environment.

   ▸ In an open system, input and output from both the internal and external environment are free-flowing.

FIGURE 8-1.
MAP OF SYSTEMS THEORY

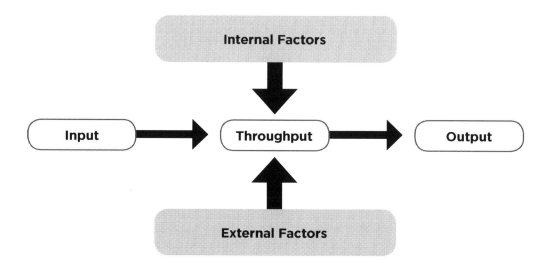

System Components

As delineated in *Nursing Professional Development: Scope & Standards of Practice* (ANA & NNSDO, 2010, pp. 3–9), systems components of nursing professional development as specialized nursing practice are:

▶ Input

　▷ Learner

　　▷ Individual or group with an educational need

　▷ Nursing professional development specialist is a registered nurse with expertise in nursing education who

　　▷ Demonstrates standards of the nursing professional development specialist

　　▷ Supports lifelong learners

　　▷ Fosters learning and creates an appropriate climate for learning

▶ Throughputs (process)

　▷ Evidence-based practice

　　▷ Core of the nursing professional development system

　　▷ Integration of best practice, research, educational and clinical expertise, and learner values

　▷ Practice-based evidence

　　▷ Study methodology that relates more directly to practice effectiveness and improvement

　　▷ Uses practice-to-science model to identify most effective practice

　▷ Orientation

　　▷ Educational process of introducing new staff or students to an organization or department

　　▷ Also implemented when roles, responsibilities, or practices change

　▷ Competency program

　　▷ Establishes expected level of performance for a group of activities

　　▷ Nursing professional development specialist possesses expertise in competency assessment and its development, facilitation, implementation, and evaluation of competency programs

- Inservice education

    - Learning in the work setting to assist staff in performing their work duties

    - Includes learning about policy and procedure changes or use of new products

- Continuing education

    - Systematic professional learning designed to augment knowledge, skills, and attitude

    - Three types of learning modalities: provider-directed, learner-directed, and learner-paced

- Career development and role transition

    - Assists the learner in identifying and developing strategies for achieving career goals throughout the nurse's lifetime

- Research and scholarship

    - Conducts, encourages, disseminates, and participates in research and scholarship

    - Work environment of the nursing professional development specialist influences level of involvement

    - Applies scientific process and research results

- Academic partnership

    - Establishes mutually beneficial partnerships between academic and healthcare institutions

    - Serves as a liaison for the academic institution, which may include teaching, coordinating, and advising learners

► Outputs

- Change

    - Adapting to new behaviors and process

- Learning

    - Acquisition of knowledge, skills, abilities, and attitude for base practice

    - Influenced by various internal and external factors

- Professional role competency and growth

    - Advancement in professional growth from Benner's stages of novice through expert

    - Attainment of specialty certifications

    - Becoming nursing professional development specialist

- ▶ Environment
  - ◈ Learner
    - ▷ Any context where learning occurs
    - ▷ May overlap with practice environment and not be limited to a classroom setting
  - ◈ Nursing professional development specialist
    - ▷ Structural, social, and cultural setting in which nursing occurs
    - ▷ Multidimensional and subject to local, state, regional, national, and international regulations, initiatives, and trends
    - ▷ Depends on material and human resources within the practice
    - ▷ Promotes transformational leadership
    - ▷ Supports nursing collaborative relationship with other disciples and academic partnerships
  - ◈ The educational and clinical environments may overlap
- ▶ System feedback
  - ◈ Feedback provides for continuous lifelong learning and growth.
  - ◈ The feedback influences the evolving practice of both nursing and nursing professional development.
  - ◈ The nursing professional development specialist uses all components of the throughput process to influence the change to the output.
- ▶ Systems theory allows for an analytical approach to the process.
  - ◈ Creates a workable framework for planning, implementing, and evaluating a process, which may be nursing education, LEAN (see Chapter 20 section on Process Improvement Methodologies), shared governance, and so on
  - ◈ Examples of other systems theory
    - ▷ Nursing process
    - ▷ Watson's theory of caring
    - ▷ Orem's theory of self-care
    - ▷ Roy's adaptation theory

Utilizing Systems Theory

▶ Nursing professional development (NPD) specialists use a conceptual approach to translate new knowledge into clinical practice.

  ▹ New information is the *input*.

  ▹ *Throughput* is the information being received by the student.

    ▷ Communication is essential.

    ▷ NPD specialists send messages.

    ▷ Students receive messages.

  ▹ Each educational situation has both internal and external factors.

    ▷ The student is affected by the social aspects and communication.

    ▷ The nursing professional development specialist role is to focus on experiences that are conducive to positive encounters.

    ▷ Interaction between the student and nursing professional development specialist is important. Every experience, including simulation, helps prepare the student for real situations in the future.

  ▹ Translation of education to clinical practice is the output. The output of a nursing education program looks at the success and effectiveness of clinical practice.

  ▹ Use of ongoing feedback mechanisms provides nursing professional development specialists with information to employ correcting measures to achieve optimal patient care.

Nursing Professional Development Role With Systems Theory

▶ Systems theory lets nursing professional development specialists implement education leading to evidence-based practice.

▶ NPD specialist's role

  ▹ Education is lifelong learning; goal is to provide education that enhances clinical effectiveness.

  ▹ Knowledge of systems theory (input, throughputs, output, and interrelationships between factors) allows the NPD specialist to modify clinical practices based on evidence and elevates professional practice standards.

  ▹ Focus on throughput processes that promote effective communication, interaction, and systems thinking.

  ▹ Outlined in the *Nursing Professional Development: Scope and Standards of Practice* (system diagram; ANA & NNSDO, 2010, p. 3).

ASSESSMENT

Learning Needs Assessment

▶ *Learning needs assessment* is a process for identifying a discrepancy between what is desired and what exists (ANCC, 2013).

▶ Needs assessment may be formal or informal.

▶ Needs assessments provide data that are used to prioritize learning needs, determine the target audience, and distinguish learning needs from systems or performance problems (Avillion, 2008; Cooper, 2002).

▶ Data are collected from a variety of sources, including

» Nurses, other employees, management, administration

▷ Patients

» Standards of accrediting organizations

» Standards of professional organizations

» Nurse practice acts

▷ Legislative rules and regulations

▷ Licensure requirements

» Job descriptions and performance evaluations

▷ Professional networks

» Nursing or healthcare literature

▷ Quality improvement data

▷ Program evaluation data (ANCC, 2013; Avillion, 2008; Shelton, 2002)

▶ Data may be collected using various strategies, such as questionnaires; surveys; interviews; focus groups; records; reports; program evaluations; tests; reviewing trends in literature, law, and healthcare; and observations (ANCC, 2013; Kitchie, 2008).

▶ Data about identified needs are documented in a manner that is retrievable and useful for all aspects of the program planning process (ANA & NNSDO, 2010).

▶ The target audience is the "group for which an educational activity has been designed" (ANCC, 2013, p. 105).

▶ The nursing professional development specialist should learn as much as possible about the target audience, including their backgrounds, levels of experience, preferred learning styles, motivation to learn, and availability to attend the activity (Bulmer, 2002).

▶ Steps in conducting a needs assessment:

 ▹ Establish the purpose.

 ▹ Identify the target audience.

 ▹ Decide who will assist with the process.

 ▹ Select a method.

 ▹ Conduct the needs assessment.

▶ Analyze and share the results with NPD specialists and other stakeholders (Cooper, 2002)

Needs Assessment Strategies

▶ Questionnaires and surveys

 ▹ Purpose: To gather information about respondents' opinions rather than objective knowledge or skills.

 ▹ Instruments may be designed with closed-ended questions (e.g., rating scales, multiple choice, Likert scale) or open-ended format (e.g., sentence-completion, completely unstructured) in written or electronic form.

 ▹ Advantages: Can collect information from a large number of respondents in a relatively short time; most learners are familiar with this type of format; forms can be completed anonymously, encouraging honest opinions; if closed-ended questions are used, data are easily tabulated and analyzed.

 ▹ Disadvantages: Possibility of low response rate; learners may not understand items; no opportunity to clarify vague or ambiguous items or responses; open-ended questions may be time-consuming to analyze (Gooding, 2013; Kitchie, 2008).

▶ Interviews

 ▹ Purpose: To provide for in-depth discussion of learning needs and areas of concern.

 ▹ Interviews may be structured (specific sequence of direct, focused questions) or unstructured (general question with follow-up).

 ▹ Advantages: More in-depth, thorough responses, especially if rapport established; responses can be clarified with follow-up questions.

 ▹ Disadvantages: Information subjectively interpreted by the interviewer; interviewees may provide responses that they think the interviewer wants to hear; responses, especially in unstructured interview, may be difficult to objectively analyze (Gooding, 2013; Kitchie, 2008)

▶ Focus groups

> ▹ Purpose: To provide for in-depth discussion about a specific learning need or topic.

> ▹ A focus group consists of 4 to 12 potential learners who participate in a 60- to 90-minute discussion.

> ▹ A facilitator leads the discussion by asking open-ended questions that encourage dialogue.

> ▹ An observer is present to take notes or record the discussion with permission of the participants.

> ▹ Advantages: Source of rich qualitative data about specific learning needs; conveys sense of value for learners' ideas and opinions.

> ▹ Disadvantages: Participants may feel some reluctance to honestly express ideas; may be time-consuming to analyze (Cooper, 2002; Gooding, 2013; Kitchie, 2008)

▶ Records and reports

> ▹ Purpose: To gather information from existing data sources that may illustrate learning needs.

> ▹ Examples of reports that are commonly used to assess learning needs include quality improvement reports and audits, patient record audits, infection control reports, event reports, annual reports, and patient surveys.

> ▹ Records that provide needs assessment data may include program evaluation summaries, meeting minutes, position descriptions, and performance appraisals.

> ▹ Advantages: Process and tools are already in place and readily accessible; identified learning needs relate to organizational priorities.

> ▹ Disadvantages: Findings may reflect organizational system needs rather than individual learning needs; may be time-consuming to analyze (Cooper, 2002; Yoder Wise, 1996)

▶ Tests

> ▹ Purpose: To assess knowledge and skill levels on a specific topic to identify gaps and tailor teaching to meet learning needs.

> ▹ Testing is complex. The test developer must use a test blueprint and consider validity, reliability, pilot testing, and criterion or norm-referenced grading. (See Chapter 9 for more information on test development.)

> ▹ Advantages: Findings helpful to tailor educational plan to specific audience.

> ▹ Disadvantages: Data may reflect problems with test-taking ability rather than learning needs; time-consuming to develop a valid and reliable testing tool (Kitchie, 2008; Yoder Wise, 1996).

▶ Observations

» Purpose: To validate data from other sources and determine discrepancies between stated behavior and actual behavior.

» Observations may be planned or incidental.

» Specific standards must be used to observe behavior, and observed behaviors must be documented using a checklist or other form of documentation.

» If multiple observers are involved, interrater reliability must be determined.

» Advantages: Provide information about actual values and performance rather than reported values and performance; excellent source of information about needs related to performance of skills.

» Disadvantages: Person being observed may alter behaviors if he or she knows observation is occurring; time-consuming for observer (Gooding, 2013).

▶ When possible, needs assessment data should be validated using more than one data collection method (e.g., gap identified in infection control data confirmed through staff survey; Shelton, 2002).

▶ The nursing professional development specialist objectively analyzes data from multiple sources (e.g., survey, event report, administrative mandate) to determine learning needs before developing an educational plan.

▶ The nursing professional development specialist involves key stakeholders in prioritizing learning needs based on factors such as organizational goals, available financial and staff resources, and the significance of the need to patient care (Cooper, 2002; Shelton, 2002).

PLANNING

General Principles

▶ The educational planning process involves development of a clear purpose or goal statement and measurable objectives that are appropriate for the target audience, content, teaching methods, and evaluation strategies.

▶ A *purpose*, often referred to as a learning goal, is a written outcome statement about what the learner will be able to do at the conclusion of the activity (i.e., "The purpose of this activity is to enable the learner to…"; ANCC, 2013).

▶ *Behavioral objectives* are based on identified learning needs.

　▹ Behavioral objectives clearly state the learner outcomes of an educational activity in specific and measurable terms (Bastable & Doody, 2008).

▶ Content for an educational activity is congruent with the activity's purpose and educational objectives.

▶ Teaching and learning strategies are congruent with the activity's objectives and content.

▶ The nursing professional development specialist defines a clear method that includes learner input to evaluate the effectiveness of an educational activity (ANCC, 2013).

Writing Behavioral Objectives

▶ The principles of adult learning are incorporated in the development of educational objectives.

▶ Objectives are written in behavioral terms appropriate to the target audience and specifically identify what the learner must accomplish.

▶ Each objective contains only one expected behavior.

▶ Behavioral objectives describe learner outcomes in the cognitive, psychomotor, or affective domains of learning. (See Chapter 4 for information on the domains of learning.)

▶ Objectives must contain an action verb that explicitly identifies in observable and measurable terms what the learner must do to successfully complete the learning activity.

▶ Well-written objectives include four components that can be represented by the acronym ABCD:

　▹ **Audience:** Identifies the learner as the focus (who)

　▹ **Behavior:** Action that the learner will be able to do to demonstrate that learning has occurred (what)

　▹ **Condition:** The circumstances under which the learner is expected to perform the actions (how)

　▹ **Degree of attainment:** The standard (e.g., accuracy, timing, amount) to which actions must conform to be acceptable (how well; Bastable & Doody, 2008; Bruce, 2002)

▶ Sample objectives for each domain of learning

    ▹ Cognitive: After completing a self-learning module (C), the learner (A) is able to explain (B) the action of three chemotherapeutic agents (D) used in the treatment of breast cancer.

    ▹ Psychomotor: Given a selection of dressing supplies (C), the learner (A) is able to demonstrate (B) a sterile dressing change following the institutional guideline (D).

    ▹ Affective: Following a facilitated group discussion (C), the learner (A) is able to implement (B) three strategies for overcoming barriers to caring for patients from other cultures (D).

Content Determination

▶ *Content* is the subject matter of an educational activity and is "reflective of the stated objectives and evidence-based practice" (ANA & NNSDO, 2010, p. 26).

▶ Content is individualized to the target audience, according to the participants' basic and advanced education, experience, and preferred learning style.

▶ The nursing professional development specialist collaborates with members of the target audience and content experts to develop content for an educational activity based on the best available evidence (ANA & NNSDO, 2010; ANCC, 2013).

▶ Content is developed in a cost-efficient manner using available resources.

▶ Content is organized in a logical and meaningful sequence, congruent with the activity's learning objectives.

▶ Content may be structured to present general concepts followed by specific examples, simple to complex, theoretical principles to practical application, chronological order, or some other logical flow of information (DeYoung, 2009; Leroux & Cody, 1996).

Selection of Faculty and Content Experts

▶ Faculty and content experts must have credible experience and expertise in the content to be presented.

▶ Faculty must have knowledge of the educational process, including principles of adult learning and learning styles.

▶ Faculty must use an informative, engaging presentation style that encourages participation, addresses participant questions, and incorporates techniques that are appropriate to the objectives.

▶ Faculty must be comfortable presenting content using the teaching format identified (e.g., distance learning, videotape).

▶ Content experts must use current expertise and an evidence-based approach to develop content for independent study modules and other types of learner-paced activities.

▶ Faculty and content experts may be identified from within or outside the organization (Bulmer, 2002).

   ▷ Experts from within the organization

      ▷ Know the organizational culture, goals, and objectives

      ▷ Know and are known to the target audience

      ▷ May be expected to present educational activities as part of their role

      ▷ May not be able to bring unique or external perspectives to the audience

   ▷ Experts external to the organization

      ▷ Bring a unique or external perspective to an educational activity

      ▷ May be perceived as more prestigious than internal presenters

      ▷ Require a contract or letter of agreement outlining needs and expenses

      ▷ May be unaware of organizational culture, goals, and objectives

Selection of Teaching Strategies

▶ *Teaching strategies* include the "instructional methods and techniques that are in accord with principles of adult learning" (ANCC, 2013, p. 106).

▶ A variety of teaching strategies may be necessary to promote learning in adults who have different backgrounds, experience, and learning style preferences (O'Shea, 2002).

▶ The nursing professional development specialist selects teaching strategies after considering several factors, including

   ▷ Adult learning principles

   ▷ Audience characteristics (e.g., group size, diversity, level of expertise)

   ▷ Educator's expertise and preferences for teaching strategies

   ▷ Learning objectives

   ▷ Complexity of content

   ▷ Cost-effectiveness

   ▷ Setting for educational activity

   ▷ Time

   ▷ Available resources (e.g., technology aids, materials, manikins; Fitzgerald, 2008)

▶ Clark (2008) identified four qualities of teaching methods to consider when teaching.

    1. Fidelity means that the strategy closely aligns in realism to the actual situation.

    2. Cost refers to the expense of a teaching strategy.

    3. Safety can be applied to the patient (e.g., risk of harm) or the learner (e.g., negative experience).

    4. Completeness means that the strategy provides practice opportunities that may not be immediately available in the real world.

Description of Teaching Strategies

▶ Lecture

    ▹ Structured method in which the presenter uses a prepared oral presentation to give new information to groups of learners

    ▹ Useful when a large amount of information must be presented to large groups

    ▹ Limited flexibility in scheduling or delivery of content

    ▹ More effective if opportunities for interaction and feedback are incorporated by combining lecture with small group discussion, group exercises, question-and-answer sessions, audiovisual aids, or other interactive strategies (Aucoin, 1998; Fitzgerald, 2008; Rowles & Russo, 2009)

▶ Group discussion

    ▹ Method of teaching whereby learners exchange information and opinions with one another and the presenter

    ▹ Useful for problem-solving, exploring attitudes, sharing information, and critique of concepts when participants have some knowledge of topic

    ▹ May want to incorporate visual or hands-on activities to involve more than the auditory sense

    ▹ Allows for clarification of information, response to questions, and discussion of concerns

    ▹ Less faculty control and structure (Fitzgerald, 2008; Gianella, 1996)

▶ Demonstration

  ▹ Most frequently used for psychomotor skills

  ▹ Engages the learner through stimulation of visual, auditory, and tactile senses

  ▹ Often used in combination with return demonstration to validate learner achievement of objectives

  ▹ Requires adequate time, ample equipment, and small group size to provide opportunity for practice and supervision (Fitzgerald, 2008; Rowles & Russo, 2009)

▶ Role play

  ▹ Experiential learning method in which learners participate in a dramatization of a real work situation or a case study

  ▹ Often used to achieve objectives in the affective domain but may be used for cognitive and psychomotor domain objectives

  ▹ Learners may volunteer or be assigned to a defined role in the situation

  ▹ Useful to enhance problem-solving and critical thinking skills

  ▹ Best done in small groups in a nonthreatening environment to encourage participation and active involvement

  ▹ Debriefing occurs at the conclusion of the dramatization (Clark, 2008; Fitzgerald, 2008; O'Shea, 2002)

▶ Simulation

  ▹ Experiential learning method in which a clinical situation is replicated in accuracy and detail in a safe environment

  ▹ Used to teach cognitive, psychomotor, and affective domains

  ▹ May be done using written scenarios, videotape, models, actors, peers, or high-fidelity manikins

  ▹ Allows for realistic learner involvement in managing or responding to a clinical situation as an individual or as a member of a team

  ▹ Useful when situation occurs infrequently in the clinical setting or when learning in the actual work setting may compromise patient safety or is ethically or legally questionable

  ▹ Debriefing occurs at the conclusion of the simulation (Fitzgerald, 2008; Gianella, 1996)

▶ Gaming

   ▹ Experiential learning method in which learners apply knowledge and skills as they participate in a structured, competitive activity

   ▹ Used primarily for cognitive domain but may be used to supplement skills and behavior in psychomotor and affective domains

   ▹ Effective for review or reinforcement of content

   ▹ May be designed for individual or team use

   ▹ May be fun but must contribute to achievement of learning objectives

   ▹ Competitive environment may be threatening to some learners

   ▹ Debriefing occurs at the conclusion of the game to highlight key concepts (Fitzgerald, 2008; Gianella, 1996; O'Shea, 2002; Rowles & Russo, 2009)

▶ Posters

   ▹ Visual representation of concepts to convey information

   ▹ Colorful, visually stimulating format to convey detailed information in a concise way

   ▹ Allows learner to review information at a comfortable pace

   ▹ Useful to share procedural or process information or visual content (Aucoin, 1998; Rowles & Russo, 2009)

▶ Self-learning modules

   ▹ Packets of materials designed for independent study of a specific topic at the learner's pace

   ▹ Faculty serves as a facilitator and resource to the learner

   ▹ Used primarily for learning in the cognitive domain and the psychomotor domain if learning objectives include application to practice

   ▹ Alternative to traditional methods when learners are not readily able to leave the work unit for a class

   ▹ Effective for self-directed learners who are self-disciplined to complete the required work in a timely manner

   ▹ May include various learning media such as articles, handouts, web pages, audiovisuals, and equipment displays (Aucoin, 1998; Fitzgerald, 2008; Gianella, 1996; O'Shea, 2002)

▶ Computer-assisted instruction

  ▹ Delivery of educational content electronically

  ▹ Used primarily to promote learning in the cognitive domain

  ▹ May be in the form of computer or web-based presentations, tutorials, drill and practice, simulations, or testing

  ▹ Requires funding to develop or purchase

  ▹ If not web-based, limited opportunity for interaction with other learners or NPD specialists

  ▹ Must have adequate technological knowledge or support to implement and use effectively (Bowman, 2002; Clark, 2008; DeYoung, 2009; Hainsworth, 2008)

▶ Case studies and grand rounds

  ▹ Analysis and application of theoretical content to a real situation

  ▹ Used effectively to reinforce theoretical content by presenting complex situations requiring application of content using problem-solving and critical thinking

  ▹ Case study must be well designed case study to achieve learning objectives

  ▹ Most effective in an open, nonthreatening, interactive learning environment

  ▹ Link between theoretical and practical content encourages retention of important information (Aucoin, 1998; Rowles & Russo, 2009)

▶ Learning contract

  ▹ Individualized written or verbal agreement between faculty and student that describes what the learner must do to achieve learning objectives, what resources faculty provides, and criteria that will be used to determine success

  ▹ Identifies behavioral objectives to be achieved, instructional strategies and resources, method of evaluation of objective achievement, and target dates for completion

  ▹ Empowers the learner because contract development emphasizes self-direction and negotiation for learning activities and outcomes

  ▹ Actively involves the learner at all stages of the educational process from learning needs assessment through evaluation (Bastable & Doody, 2008; DeYoung, 2009)

▶ Others

  ▹ Many other strategies or variations of those listed above are available.

  ▹ Some of these include debate, role-modeling, storytelling, online forum, and videoconference

IMPLEMENTATION

General Principles

▶ According to Standard 5 of *Nursing Professional Development: Scope and Standards of Practice*, the nursing professional development specialist "implements the plan in a safe and timely manner" (ANA & NNSDO, 2010, p. 27).

▶ In addition, in the same document Standard 15 of Professional Performance states "the nursing professional development specialist considers factors related to safety, effectiveness, and cost in regard to professional development activities and expected outcomes" (ANA & NNSDO, 2010, p. 41).

▶ See Chapter 9 for information pertaining to design and delivery skills.

EVALUATION

Outcomes

▶ An *outcome* is "something that follows, is the result of, or is the consequence of a project, program, or event" (ANA & NNSDO, 2010, p. 45).

▶ Outcomes usually involve a change in knowledge, competence, practice, or patient care.

▶ Learning outcomes are identified by the behavioral objectives and are consistent with the educational activity's purpose and teaching strategies.

▶ The evaluation process measures the achievement of learning outcomes in relation to the intended learning outcomes (Kirkpatrick & DeWitt, 2009; Webb, 2002).

▶ See Chapter 11 for a discussion of types and models of evaluation as well as uses of evaluative data.

REFERENCES

American Nurses Association and National Nursing Staff Development Organization (2010). *Nursing professional development: Scope and standards of practice.* Silver Spring, MD: Nursesbooks.org.

American Nurses Credentialing Center. (2013). 2013 *ANCC primary accreditation application manual for providers and approvers.* Silver Spring, MD: Author.

Aucoin, J. W. (1998). Program planning: Solving the problem. In K. J. Kelly-Thomas, *Clinical and nursing staff development: Current competence, future focus* (2nd ed., pp. 213–239). Philadelphia: Lippincott.

Avillion, A. E. (2008). *A practical guide to staff development: Evidence-based tools and techniques for effective education* (2nd ed.). Marblehead, MA: HCPro.

Bastable, S. B., & Doody, J. A. (2008). Behavioral objectives. In S. B. Bastable (Ed.), *Nurse as educator: Principles of teaching and learning for nursing practice* (3rd ed., pp. 383–427). Boston: Jones & Bartlett.

Bowman, K. R. (2002). Using computers in education. In K. L. O'Shea, *Staff development nursing secrets* (pp. 139–147). Philadelphia: Hanley & Belfus.

Bruce, S. L. (2002). Writing objectives. In B. E. Puetz & J. W. Aucoin (Eds.), *Conversations in nursing professional development* (pp. 139–150). Pensacola, FL: Pohl Publishing.

Bulmer, J. M. (2002). Program planning. In K. L. O'Shea, *Staff development nursing secrets* (pp. 79–93). Philadelphia: Hanley & Belfus.

Clark, C. C. (2008). *Classroom skills for nurse educators.* Sudbury, MA: Jones & Bartlett

Cooper, D. C. (2002). Needs assessment. In K. L. O'Shea. *Staff development nursing secrets* (pp. 65–78). Philadelphia: Hanley & Belfus.

DeYoung, S. (2009). *Teaching strategies for nurse educators* (2nd ed.). Upper Saddle River, NJ: Prentice Hall.

Fitzgerald, K. (2008). Instructional methods and settings. In S. B. Bastable (Ed.), *Nurse as educator: Principles of teaching and learning for nursing practice* (3rd ed., pp. 429–471). Boston: Jones & Bartlett.

Gianella, A. (1996). Effective teaching and learning strategies for adults. In R. S. Abruzzese (Ed.), *Nursing staff development: Strategies for success* (2nd ed., pp. 223–241). St. Louis, MO: Mosby.

Gooding, N. (2013). Learning needs assessment. In S. L. Bruce (Ed.), *Core curriculum for nursing professional development* (4th ed., pp. 181–195). Chicago: Association for Nursing Professional Development.

Green, D. A. (2013). Educational planning. In S. L. Bruce (Ed.), *Core curriculum for nursing professional development* (4th ed., pp. 197–221). Chicago: Association for Nursing Professional Development.

Hainsworth, D. S. (2008). Instructional materials. In S. B. Bastable (Ed.), *Nurse as educator: Principles of teaching and learning for nursing practice* (3rd ed., pp. 473–514). Boston: Jones & Bartlett.

Kirkpatrick, J. M., & DeWitt, D. A. (2009). Strategies for assessing/evaluating learning outcomes. In D. M. Billings & J. A. Halstead (Eds.), *Teaching in nursing: A guide for faculty* (3rd ed., pp. 409–428). St. Louis, MO: Saunders.

Kitchie, S. (2008). Determinants of learning. In S. B. Bastable (Ed.), *Nurse as educator: Principles of teaching and learning for nursing practice* (3rd ed., pp. 93–145). Boston: Jones & Bartlett.

Leroux, D. S., & Cody, B. (1996). Curriculum planning and development. In R. S. Abruzzese (Ed.), *Nursing staff development: Strategies for success.* (2nd ed., pp. 209–222). St. Louis, MO: Mosby.

O'Shea, K. L. (2002). *Staff development nursing secrets.* Philadelphia: Hanley & Belfus.

Rowles, C. J., & Russo, B. L. (2009). Strategies to promote critical thinking and active learning. In D. M. Billings & J. A. Halstead (Eds.), *Teaching in nursing: A guide for faculty* (3rd ed., pp. 238–261). St. Louis, MO: Saunders.

Shelton, D. P. (2002). Assessing learning needs. In B. E. Puetz & J. W. Aucoin (Eds.), *Conversations in nursing professional development* (pp. 133–137). Pensacola, FL: Pohl Publishing.

Webb, D. G. (2002). Evaluating. In B. E. Puetz & J. W. Aucoin (Eds.), *Conversations in nursing professional development* (pp. 177–183). Pensacola, FL: Pohl Publishing.

Yoder Wise, P. S. (1996). Learning needs assessment. In R. S. Abruzzese (Ed.), *Nursing staff development: Strategies for success* (2nd ed., pp.188–207). St. Louis, MO: Mosby Inc.

CHAPTER 9

DESIGN AND DELIVERY SKILLS

PRESENTATION SKILLS

Preparation

▶ Know the audience; address their needs.

▶ Select content based on learning objectives.

▶ Define the purpose; the lecture method is not appropriate for all content.

▶ Organize the information:

  » Simple to complex

  » According to issues

  » According to a timeline

  » Tell them what you are going to tell them, tell them, tell them what you told them.

▶ Use an outline to assist with a logical presentation with clear connections.

▶ Presentation components:

  » Introduction that captures audience's attention

  » Three to five core messages in the body of the talk

  » Conclusion that focuses on a call to action, an inspiration, or a summary

▶ Content is current and evidence-based.

▶ Anticipate audience questions, have answers prepared or incorporated into content.

▶ Practice with one or several people who will give you constructive feedback (Paterson, 2002; Vollman, 2005).

Delivery

▶ Avoid alcohol and difficult-to-digest foods the night before a presentation.

▶ A prespeech warm-up can consist of affirming, breathing, and composing oneself.

▶ Start with a powerful introduction to capture attention within the first 90 seconds.

▶ Maintain eye contact throughout the presentation.

▶ Strengthen message using "hooks" (e.g., humor, analogies, personal experiences).

▶ Use body language and voice to emphasize points.

▶ Change from lecture to another teaching strategy (e.g., asking audience to share, using audio or video clips) every 10 to 20 minutes to hold audience attention.

▶ Do not read verbatim from notes.

▶ Do not turn back to audience to read from slides.

▶ Be prepared to delete a section if low on time or add a section if there is time left.

▶ Use the question-and-answer period to reinforce key messages (Paterson, 2002; Vollman, 2005).

Motivating Participants and Keeping Their Attention

▶ Create a positive and interesting environment for learners to motivate themselves.

▶ Recognize the value of the learners.

▶ Involve learners in the educational process.

▶ Gain learners' commitment by asking them what they want to gain in the class.

▶ Vary the teaching methods every 10 to 20 minutes.

▶ Use activities that require physical movement to teach or reinforce the message (Deck, 2002).

▶ Use the Attention, Relevance, Confidence, and Satisfaction (ARCS) Model of Motivational Design:

  » Sustain listeners' interest and curiosity (Attention)

  » Make presentation relevant and satisfying (Relevance)

  » Instill confidence; success encourages the learner to proceed (Confidence)

  » Leave satisfied after a learning goal has been achieved (Satisfaction; Paterson, 2002)

Tips to Help Learning

- ▶ Content makes sense.

- ▶ Content is related to the role of the learner.

- ▶ Content can be realistically applied.

- ▶ Content is presented in manageable increments.

- ▶ The presenter has credibility.

- ▶ The presentation is lively.

- ▶ Potential obstacles to implementation are addressed.

- ▶ Opportunities exist for implementation of new or reinforced knowledge and skills.

- ▶ Opportunities exist for reflection on the implementation process.

- ▶ The learner is continually challenged to grow (Dickerson, 2003).

IMAGES AND HANDOUTS

Images

- ▶ Need to be visible by participants

- ▶ Must add to content, not be merely decorative

- ▶ Make the message easier for the learner

- ▶ Focus participant attention to one place

- ▶ Avoid images and graphics that are not related to the content

- ▶ Consider copyright issues related to images (see Chapter 5 for discussion of copyright considerations)

Handouts

- ▶ Used for participant to follow along; however, allows participant to also look ahead.

- ▶ Include a content outline of the major concepts.

- ▶ Keep to a maximum of 10 pages.

- ▶ Can include the "nice to know" that is not covered due to time limitations.

- ▶ Include graphs, charts, and so on from visuals.

- ▶ Handouts must be clear, clean copies and typed, never handwritten.

- ▶ When handouts are produced from electronic slides (e.g., PowerPoint), ensure all content can be read in the smaller printed format.

▶ Do not reproduce copyrighted material without written permission from the copyright holder.

▶ Handouts may be enhanced with illustrations, but do not overwhelm the reader with too much color or "action."

▶ Preprinted educational material is available from third parties (Avillion, 2008).

Flip Charts

▶ Flip charts can be especially useful for group activities, focus groups, and problem-solving activities.

▶ Limit information on each page to avoid confusion.

▶ Use dark colors and print in capital letters to enhance visibility.

▶ Flip-chart content can be prepared ahead or added during the presentation.

▶ Completed pages can be posted in the room for later reference.

▶ Flip-chart paper is available plain or with lines or grids, and with or without removable adhesive.

▶ May need to flip back and forth to previous sheets.

▶ Flip charts are not feasible for large audiences due to size limitation (Misko, 2013).

Electronic Slides

▶ Present one main concept on each slide.

▶ Include information on slides to support and reinforce key concepts.

▶ Use key words and phrases, not sentences.

▶ Use a maximum of six lines per slide and six words per line.

▶ Avoid using multicolored backgrounds, which compete with written words and make them hard to distinguish.

▶ The greater the contrast between text and background color, the easier to see for participant.

▶ A lighter background with dark text may be more visible in a well-lit room, while lighter text on a dark background works better in a dimly lit room.

▶ Do not use more than two different font styles.

▶ Sans serif fonts (e.g., Arial) are easier for the eye to see on a computer or projection screen; serif fonts (e.g., Times New Roman) are easier for the eye to follow on paper where lines of text are longer.

▶ The font size should be at least 24 point; check projection in the room for readability from the farthest seat.

▶ Avoid all capitals, italics, and low-contrast font colors because these are difficult for the eye to read. For emphasis use bold, shadowing, different font color, or place text within a shape (e.g., oval, box).

▶ Keep bullets and slide transitions consistent throughout presentation.

▶ Do not overwhelm the viewer with moving objects and slide animation; use these features only when they enhance or reinforce content and not simply for variety.

▶ Use sound effects, music, etc., to enhance, not compete with, written concepts.

▶ Include graphs, charts, and demographics as part of the handout in addition to including them in the computer presentation.

▶ Use visuals in addition to text whenever possible.

▶ When embedding video clips or Internet links, verify before the presentation that they work with the set-up to be used.

▶ While electronic slides load faster when on the computer's hard drive, always bring a back-up copy.

▶ Electronic slides are portable and easily updated, reorganized, and stored (Paradi, 2003; Wilkinson, 2002).

Flyers

▶ Flyers are typically used to alert internal staff of upcoming educational activities.

▶ Information to include on flyers: name of program, dates, times, location, and target audience.

▶ Include the purpose of the program, the speaker, and if contact hours are available to pique interest of potential attendees.

▶ Lay information out clearly, providing enough white space for ease of readability.

▶ Use of attractive colors is eye-catching; be sure contrast between colors does not reduce readability.

▶ Proofread to avoid errors, especially in date, time, and location (Bodin, 2009).

Simulation

▶ Simulation is a good tool for nursing professional development (NPD) specialists to use to accelerate the progress of nurses from novices to experts.

▶ Simulation provides a safe way for a novice practitioner to practice skills in physical assessment, psychomotor skills development, and communication techniques without jeopardizing or inconveniencing patients.

▶ Simulation has been used in medical education for centuries. Examples include

  » Live patients

  » Use of medical cadavers

  » IV or phlebotomy arm

  » Injection or suture practice pads

  » Resusci Anne®

  » Advanced computerized patient simulators

▶ Clinical simulation is designed to bridge the gap between knowledge gained in the classroom and clinical practice with patients.

▶ Patient simulation has been instituted to enhance patient safety.

Fidelity Simulation

▶ *Fidelity* describes how a simulation mimics real patient interactions. The level of fidelity depends on the educational outcome of learning a psychomotor skill or integration of complex skills and critical thinking.

▶ *High-fidelity simulation* uses a computerized manikin that mimics physiological and anatomical responses to therapeutic procedures and medications according to mathematical models (Healey, Sherbino, Fan, Mensour, Upahye, & Wast, 2010).

  Requires human and financial resources for use.

  Examples include SimMan® (www.laerdal.com/simman/), Harvey® (http://www.laerdal.com/us/harvey), and Medi-SIM (http://medi-sim.mobi/).

  Allows for integrating complex skills in simulated environments to replicate the real patient situations.

▶ *Low-fidelity simulations* do not require computerized equipment. The simulation can range from role-play to manikins (used with CPR equipment and SimMan).

  » Requires minimal to moderate financial resources.

  » Examples are CDs with lung sounds and IV arms.

  » Focus on integration of psychomotor skills or a component of the real patient situation.

▶ Feedback regarding performance is the single most important feature of simulation-based learning. At the completion of the simulation (high or low), the learner should be provided with feedback regarding whether the objectives were achieved.

▶ Nursing professional development specialists need to consider many aspects when choosing simulation: educational outcomes, characteristics of the learner and instructor, space, and financial resources.

▶ Effective simulation can be achieved with both low- and high-fidelity simulation.

   ▷ High fidelity is not necessarily better than low fidelity.

   ▷ Reflection during the debriefing process is a critical element component because this is where learning occurs. Students synthesize the experience, have the opportunity to share, and discuss the experience, all of which improves clinical reasoning or critical thinking skills.

   ▷ To identify the best level of simulation needed, the critical task being instructed should be broken down into elements. Simulation for each element is then defined.

   ▷ The goal of simulation is to ensure effective transfer of knowledge to real patients.

USE OF TECHNOLOGY

▶ Technology addresses adult learning principles by meeting individual learning styles, providing interactivity, and offering self-paced learning.

▶ Types of technology that can be used in the learning environment include tele- and videoconferencing, webinars, computer-based training, Internet, and high-fidelity simulators.

▶ The use of these modalities is classified as *e-learning* (Bowman, 2002).

▶ Choose a technology that enhances the content; the goal is to make it easier for the learner to remember the message.

▶ When using technology, ensure visual and audio will function in the presentation room.

▶ Verify that software versions are compatible between electronic file and computer.

▶ Know how to troubleshoot technology or whom to contact for timely assistance.

▶ The nursing professional development specialist facilitates the learner's adaptation to new technology by providing instruction and practice with the technology, demonstrating the technology's relationship to improved patient care, and providing emotional support.

- ▶ The nursing professional development specialist provides assistance with computer literacy.

- ▶ E-learning can reduce the time the NPD specialist spends providing repetitive training and can augment knowledge acquisition so time in the classroom can be spent on application (Bowman, 2002).

- ▶ Computer-based training (CBT) is typically the first step into the use of technology. CBT can be purchased from vendors or developed in-house if the organization has the resources.

- ▶ Vendors who supply CBT may also provide learning management systems (LMS). An LMS may be limited to attendance records or provide a level of sophistication that allows course registration, as well as the creation of rosters, name tags, grade sheets, and reports (Bowman, 2002).

- ▶ Limitations to the use of technology include

    - ▹ High cost

    - ▹ Availability of computer resources

    - ▹ Computer literacy of learner and instructor

    - ▹ Technology failure

    - ▹ Content not appropriate for technology

- ▶ Benefits to the use of technology include

    - ▹ Rapid knowledge dissemination

    - ▹ Decrease in face-to-face training time

    - ▹ Engage participants with different learning styles

    - ▹ Flexibility with asynchronous learning (DiMauro, 2002; Gloe, 2002; Holtschneider, 2013).

TEST CONSTRUCTION

- ▶ Tests are commonly used to evaluate the cognitive domain, although a skill demonstration test can be used to evaluate the psychomotor domain.

- ▶ Tests need to be valid and reliable to ensure they are measuring the desired outcome.

    - ▹ A valid test measures what it is expected to measure.

    - ▹ A reliable test consistently yields the same, or nearly the same, score for a person taking the test several times during a span in which the trait being measured is not expected to change.

▶ The length of a test is determined by the amount of time that can be devoted to testing.

▶ Typically, a learner is given one minute for each multiple-choice question. Alternative item types may require longer times for responses (Haladyna, 1999; Kubisyn & Borich, 2000; Oermann & Gaberson, 2006).

Validity

▶ Content validity is assessed by comparing test items to learning objectives to see if they match. A test blueprint assists with this task.

▷ A test blueprint is a grid with the objectives written down the first column and the cognitive domain levels (knowledge, comprehension, application, etc.) in ascending order along the top row.

▶ The total number of test questions is divided among the objectives according to importance and each objective's cognitive domain level. The higher the cognitive level, the more questions can be asked for that objective.

▶ Questions are developed at the objective's domain level and lower. For example, if an objective is at the application level, the questions pertaining to that level are written at the application level and may include questions at the knowledge and comprehension level.

▶ The grid is filled in with the numbers of questions for each objective in each domain.

▶ The questions are then reviewed according to the test blueprint to ensure the questions address the objectives at the levels indicated.

▶ Writing test items at different cognitive levels is a learned skill and develops with practice.

▶ When using a test bank, ensure the questions align with content and domain level of the objectives (Haladyna, 1999; Kubisyn & Borich, 2000; Oermann & Gaberson, 2006).

Reliability

▶ Reliability is best determined when a test is designed to measure a single basic concept.

▶ Reliability is affected by group variability, the number of test items, and the difficulty of test items.

▶ "All tests are imperfect and are subject to error" (Kubisyn & Borich, 2000, p. 321). Therefore, it is important for the nursing professional development specialist to take steps to increase the accuracy and decrease the error of tests.

▶ These steps include

> ▷ Having distractors of the multiple choice items be plausible to the uninformed

> ▷ Ensuring that no test item is dependent on the learner's response to another question

> ▷ Removing ambiguous questions

> ▷ Writing the test at an appropriate reading level

> ▷ Having clear, specific, written directions for completing the test

> ▷ Verifying that the test answer key is correct (Haladyna, 1999; Kubisyn & Borich, 2000; Oermann & Gaberson, 2006).

Difficulty Level

▶ The purpose of the test determines the difficulty level of test items even when items are written at higher cognitive levels.

▶ If the purpose is to verify the learner has "gotten" the message, such as with mandatory training, then the goal is 100% for passing. In other words, 100% of the people responding to the question answer it correctly.

▶ If the purpose is to ensure the learner can function in a specific unit at a specific level, such as for a critical care course, then the goal may be 80% for passing. In other words, 80% of the people responding to the question answer it correctly.

▶ Review questions to determine that the distractors are plausible and not obviously incorrect answers.

▶ If a large percentage of learners select the incorrect answer, determine if the item was keyed wrong, there was an error in the question, or the teaching did not address the learning need (Haladyna, 1999; Kubisyn & Borich, 2000).

REFERENCES

Avillion, A. E. (2008). *A practical guide to staff development: Evidence-based tools and techniques for effective education* (2nd ed.). Marblehead, MA: HCPro.

Bodin, S. (2009). Marketing educational activities. In S. L. Bruce (Ed.), *Core curriculum for staff development* (3rd ed., pp. 347–360). Pensacola, FL: National Nursing Staff Development Organization.

Bowman, K. R. (2002). Using computers in education. In K. L. O'Shea, *Staff development nursing secrets* (pp. 139–147). Philadelphia: Hanley & Belfus.

Deck, M. L. (2002). Educator. In B. E. Puetz & J. W. Aucoin (Eds.), *Conversations in nursing professional development* (pp. 61–67). Pensacola, FL: Pohl Publishing.

Dickerson, P. S. (2003). Ten tips to help learning. *Journal of Nurses in Staff Development, 19,* 244–250.

DiMauro, N. M. (2002). Integrating technology choices into practice. In B. E. Puetz & J. W. Aucoin (Eds.), *Conversations in nursing professional development* (pp. 287–302). Pensacola, FL: Pohl Publishing.

Gloe, D. (2002). Teaching about computer use. In B. E. Puetz & J. W. Aucoin (Eds.), *Conversations in nursing professional development* (pp. 303–312). Pensacola, FL: Pohl Publishing.

Haladyna, T. M. (1999). *Developing and validating multiple-choice test items* (2nd ed.). Mahwah, NJ: Lawrence Erlbaum Associates.

Healey, A., Sherbino, J., Fan, J., Mensour, M., Upadhye, S., & Wasi, P. (2010). A low-fidelity simulation curriculum addresses needs identified by faculty and improves the comfort level of senior internal medicine resident physicians with inhospital resuscitation. *Critical Care Medicine, 38*(9), 1899–1903.

Holtschneider, M. E. (2013). Technology and nursing professional development. In S. L. Bruce (Ed.), *Core curriculum for staff development* (4th ed., pp. 527–545). Chicago: Association for Nursing Professional Development.

Kubisyn, T., & Borich, G. (2000). *Educational testing and measurement: Classroom application and practice* (6th ed.). New York: John Wiley & Sons.

Misko, L. (2013). Implementation of learning activities. In S. L. Bruce (Ed.), *Core curriculum for staff development* (4th ed., pp. 397–423). Chicago: Association for Nursing Professional Development.

Oermann, M. H., & Gaberson, K. B. (2006). *Evaluation and testing in nursing education* (2nd ed.). New York: Springer Publishing.

Paradi, D. (2003). *Ten secrets for using PowerPoint effectively*. Retrieved from http://www.thinkoutsidetheslide.com/articles/ten_secrets_for_using_powerpoint.htm

Paterson, B. L. (2002). Presentation skills. In K. L. O'Shea, *Staff development nursing secrets* (pp. 123–129). Philadelphia: Hanley & Belfus.

Vollman, K. M. (2005). Enhancing presentation skills for the advanced practice nurse: Strategies for success. *AACN Clinical Issues, 16*, 67–77.

Wilkinson, C. S. (2002). Implementing. In B. E. Puetz, & J. W. Aucoin (Eds.), *Conversations in nursing professional development* (pp. 157–170). Pensacola, FL: Pohl Publishing.

CHAPTER 10

MARKETING AND MANAGEMENT OF EDUCATIONAL ACTIVITIES

MARKETING EDUCATIONAL ACTIVITIES

Marketing

▶ *Marketing* focuses on effectively delivering a message to a target audience to stimulate them to take action (Wilcox & Taulli-Lasseigne, 2013).

▶ Marketing materials must be accurate, comprehensive, and appealing to the target audience (American Nurses Association [ANA] and National Nursing Staff Development Organization [NNSDO], 2010).

▶ *Internal marketing* is marketing that is directed to learners and their managers within one's own place of employment (Wilcox & Taulli-Lasseigne, 2013).

▶ *External marketing* is marketing that is directed to prospective audiences outside the sponsoring organization (Wilcox & Taulli-Lasseigne, 2013).

▶ The goal of marketing in nursing professional development is to promote educational products and services that will support the organization's strategic goals and values, meet the learning needs identified by staff, and adhere to criteria of accrediting bodies.

▶ The components of marketing are

  ▹ Completion of market analysis

  ▹ Development of a marketing plan

  ▹ Implementation of a marketing plan

  ▹ Evaluation of the plan (Wilcox & Taulli-Lasseigne, 2013)

▶ A market analysis for nursing professional development includes

   ▸ Educational needs assessment

   ▸ Characteristics of the target audience

   ▸ Assessment of inconsistencies in practice in the patient-care environment

   ▸ Understanding of trends in health care, nursing practice, social and demographic environment

   ▸ Fiscal, legislative, regulatory, and accreditation environment and factors

   ▸ Understanding of the mission, strategic goals, and objectives of the organization

   ▸ Extent of resources (Alspach, 1995; Rodriguez, 1996)

The Five "P's" of a Marketing Plan

▶ *Product* refers to the items (tangible) or services (intangible) that are offered to customers.

   ▸ Nursing professional development products may include classes, workshops, self-directed learning modules, audiovisual programs, and computer-based instruction.

   ▸ Both learners and decision-makers must desire the products.

   ▸ The nursing professional development specialist is responsible for assuring the quality of product objectives, content, and teaching strategies, regardless of whether the source of the educational product is internal or external to the organization (Rodriguez, 1996; Wilcox & Taulli-Lasseigne, 2013).

▶ *Place* is the location of the educational activity.

   ▸ Considerations in selecting an internal location include comfort, size, adequate lighting and ventilation, acoustic quality, visibility of presenter and audiovisuals, and accessibility.

   ▸ Additional considerations in selecting an external location include cost, parking availability, appropriateness of setting, adjacent facilities, and security.

   ▸ Internal locations may be a conference room or classroom on or near a work unit, skills lab, lecture hall, computer lab, or simulation center.

   ▸ External locations may be a conference or convention center, public meeting space, or hotel.

▶ *Price* refers to the cost of attendance at the educational activity.

  ▷ The pricing objective may be to generate a profit, break even, or absorb the loss.

  ▷ The organization's mission and policies as well as whether the marketing focus is internal or external may influence the pricing objective (e.g., employees attend free).

  ▷ Price is determined by the pricing objective, market considerations, and total budget.

  ▷ If a registration fee is assessed, it should be high enough to reflect that the program has educational value but not so high that it is overpriced and discourages attendance (Aucoin, 1998b).

▶ *Promotion* is the action taken to communicate information about an educational activity to the largest potential target audience in a timely manner.

  ▷ Promotion may be accomplished through brochures, fliers, emails, notices in newsletters or on bulletin boards, slogans, logos, printed or electronic catalogs, word of mouth, electronic calendars or notices, mailings, social networking sites, and public announcements.

  ▷ The availability of fiscal, material, and human resources and the scope and size of the target audience may influence the selection of promotion strategies (Alspach, 1995; Wilcox & Taulli-Lasseigne, 2013).

▶ *Participants* are the identified members of the target audience for the educational activity.

  ▷ Professional and personal characteristics of the target audience should be considered in the marketing plan.

  ▷ Information gathered over time about segments of the target audience can be useful in focusing marketing efforts for specific educational activities.

Management of the Marketing Process

▶ Marketing occurs throughout the educational planning process according to an established timeline.

▶ The nursing professional development specialist assures that all standards and criteria are met in the marketing process (e.g., use of accreditation logo and language, commercial support guidelines).

▶ Implement marketing strategies at established points during the planning process (e.g., save-the-date notice, mailings, announcements, reminders).

▶ Advertising and publicity

    ▷ Methods of internal promotion

        ▷ Colorful flyers or banner announcements

        ▷ Bulletin board displays

        ▷ Newsletter or electronic news forums

        ▷ Email notices and reminders

        ▷ Word of mouth

    ▷ Methods of external promotion

        ▷ Direct mail—brochures, calendars, or catalogs

        ▷ Advertisements—free or paid

        ▷ Word of mouth

        ▷ Websites

        ▷ Email

    ▷ Design of promotional material

        ▷ Design and information may vary for internal and external audiences.

        ▷ Information to be included: title, date, time, location, program purpose, objectives, benefits to participants, target audience, schedule, faculty information, registration information, contact hours, cost, hotel information (if necessary), travel and driving directions (if necessary), parking, disability or dietary accommodations, cancellation and refund policies, and contact information

        ▷ Design elements to consider: easy-to-read font size and typeface; dark, contrasting color on light background; adequate white space; appealing, personalized format

        ▷ Promotional materials should be proofread for accuracy, completeness, and clarity of content (Alspach, 1995; Rodriguez, 1996).

    ▷ Use of mailing lists

        ▷ Mailing lists, when used, should be current, accurate, and complete.

        ▷ Mailing lists may be developed using past participant information.

        ▷ Mailing lists may be purchased for target audience from external sources (e.g., ANA, specialty organizations, board of nursing).

▶ Evaluation of marketing plan

    ▸ Collect data related to elements of marketing plan (e.g., demographic data of participants, how participants heard about or decided to attend activity).

    ▸ Analyze marketing data to determine effectiveness of strategies (e.g., track timing of registrations with mailings, announcements; monitor website visits).

    ▸ Analyze financial data to determine effectiveness of promotional costs (e.g., percentage of revenue spent on promotion; most effective strategies in producing revenue; Alspach, 1995).

MANAGEMENT OF EDUCATIONAL ACTIVITIES

Budgeting

▶ The nursing professional development specialist coordinates all aspects of the educational process, including the use of financial resources and systems needed to implement the plan (ANA & NNSDO, 2010).

▶ Definitions

    ▸ *Operational budget* reflects the day-to-day costs of operating a staff development department, including salaries and supplies.

    ▸ *Capital budget* provides for the acquisition of major equipment used over a period of time such as manikins, video equipment, and classroom furniture (Sheridan & Frost-Hartzler, 1996).

    ▸ *Revenue* is income.

    ▸ *Expenditure* is expense.

        ▹ Direct costs are out-of-pocket expenses spent on educational activities (e.g., speaker honorarium, travel, marketing, materials).

        ▹ Indirect costs are in-house contributions such as employee salaries and benefits, space, and overhead (e.g., heat, lighting, electricity) costs.

        ▹ Fixed costs are costs that remain the same regardless of the amount of business activity (e.g., classroom furniture, speaker honorarium, audiovisual support, initial publicity).

        ▹ Variable costs are costs that vary proportionally with the amount of business activity (e.g., printing, refreshments).

    ▸ Commercial support is defined as "financial or in-kind contributions given by a commercial interest that are used to pay for all or part of the costs of a CNE activity" (ANCC, 2013, p. 22).

▶ Benefit–cost ratio analysis identifies the economic efficiency of a program in terms of the relationship between costs and benefits (in monetary terms).

   ▹ Itemize costs of the educational activity.

   ▹ Itemize benefits of the educational activity to the learner, the organization, and the patient.

   ▹ Translate costs and benefits into monetary terms.

▶ Cost-effectiveness analysis measures the efficiency of achieving outcomes in relation to costs (cost per unit of outcomes achieved).

   ▹ Define realistic, measurable objectives.

   ▹ Determine program costs.

   ▹ Measure learner outcomes to evaluate success (Sheridan & Frost-Hartzler, 1996).

▶ A budget worksheet is a helpful tool in determining the expenses and revenue associated with an educational activity.

▶ A completed budget worksheet can be used to determine registration fees for the current and future educational activities.

▶ ANCC (2013) has adapted a set of *Guidelines for Ensuring Content Integrity of Continuing Nursing Education Activities* that articulates policies for disclosure and commercial support in the planning and provision of continuing nursing education activities.

Policies

▶ The nursing professional development specialist collaborates with others to develop and implement policies that address all relevant aspects of the educational activity. Areas addressed in policy and procedure statements may include

   ▹ Registration process

   ▹ Cancellation process and fees (if any)

   ▹ Silencing cell phones and pagers

   ▹ Criteria for successful completion

   ▹ Audio- or videotaping

▶ Learners must be informed in advance of policies that may influence their decision to participate in an educational activity (Aucoin, 1998a).

Process Management

▶ Preregistration may or may not be required.

▶ If used, a preregistration process must be developed and clearly communicated to potential participants.

▶ Preregistration or registration may be managed using a written or electronic form or a learning content management system.

▶ If a fee is involved, communicate the amount and what it covers (e.g., lunch, handouts) to potential participants.

▶ Have a method to collect fees via cash, check, or credit card.

▶ Communicate the policy for cancellation to potential participants.

▶ Include registrant cancellation policies and process, including any deadlines or penalties, in program marketing materials.

▶ Have a user-friendly registration process available on site the day of the educational activity (Aucoin, 1998a).

Facility Management

▶ Select a physical environment that is comfortable for learners, appropriate for the teaching strategies being used, and supportive of the presenter's requirements (Schoenly, 1998).

▶ Factors to consider in selecting a location for an educational activity:

  ▷ Target audience: Is the activity for an internal audience or targeted to a local, regional, or national audience?

  ▷ Topic, objectives, and teaching strategies: Does the educational activity require skills practice, group work, or tables for note-taking or projects?

  ▷ Availability of audiovisual, computers, and LCD projectors, including cost and availability of technical support

  ▷ Comfortable seating arrangements and room space for the size of the group

  ▷ Adequate lighting and ventilation

  ▷ Ability to control room temperature

  ▷ Minimal background noise or distractions in adjacent areas

  ▷ Availability of restrooms and other needed conveniences

  ▷ Availability of catering services for breaks and meals, if needed

    » Requirements met for Americans with Disabilities Act (ADA)

    » Availability of space as needed to accommodate posters, displays, concurrent sessions, breaks, and meals

    » Adequate, well-lit, and safe parking areas (Aucoin, 1998b; Aucoin, 2002; Wilkinson, 2002)

▶ Additional considerations for an external conference being marketed regionally or nationally include

    » Availability and cost of overnight accommodations

    » Transportation convenience and options

    » Availability of other area attractions

▶ Once the location has been determined, arrangements and details for room set-up and clean-up must be determined (Aucoin, 1998a).

On-Site Coordination

▶ Have an adequate number of handouts and other class documents (e.g., registration forms, evaluation forms, certificates of attendance) available on site.

▶ Check availability and operation of audiovisual, computer, and other equipment prior to the start of the activity.

▶ Ensure that refreshments are delivered on time.

▶ Control environmental factors such as lighting and room temperature.

▶ If coordinating a large conference or group, arrange to have staff and volunteers available to assist with identified responsibilities (e.g., room monitor, speaker support) to ensure smooth coordination throughout the educational activity.

▶ Address participant concerns or questions with courtesy and respect.

▶ Collect evaluation data and distribute certificates of attendance.

Troubleshooting

▶ Be prepared with a backup plan in case problems arise related to any of the following situations:

    » Speaker illness or unexpected conflict

    » Audiovisual, computer, or other equipment malfunction

    » Unanticipated distractions or interruptions (e.g., construction noise in a hotel, patient care activities near a unit classroom)

REFERENCES

Alspach, J. G. (1995). *The educational process in nursing staff development.* St. Louis, MO: Mosby.

American Nurses Association and National Nursing Staff Development Organization. (2010). *Nursing professional development: Scope and standards of practice.* Silver Spring, MD: Nursesbooks.org.

American Nurses Credentialing Center. (2013). *2013 ANCC primary accreditation application manual for providers and approvers.* Silver Spring, MD: Author.

Aucoin, J. W. (1998a). *101 tips to better conferences.* Pensacola, FL: National Nursing Staff Development Organization.

Aucoin, J. W. (1998b). Program planning: Solving the problem. In K. J. Kelly-Thomas, *Clinical and nursing staff development: Current competence, future focus* (2nd ed., pp. 213–239). Philadelphia: Lippincott.

Aucoin, J. W. (2002). Planning. In B. E. Puetz & J. W. Aucoin (Eds.), *Conversations in nursing professional development* (pp. 151–155). Pensacola, FL: Pohl Publishing.

Rodriguez, L. (1996). In-house marketing of staff development programs. In R. S. Abruzzese (Ed.), *Nursing staff development: Strategies for success* (2nd ed., pp. 142–155). St. Louis, MO: Mosby.

Schoenly, L. (1998). Creating an environment of learning: An opportunity. In K. J. Kelly-Thomas, *Clinical and nursing staff development: Current competence, future focus* (2nd ed., pp. 282–300). Philadelphia: Lippincott.

Sheridan, D. R., & Frost-Hartzler, P. (1996). Documenting effectiveness: Budget and cost considerations. In R. S. Abruzzese (Ed.), *Nursing staff development: Strategies for success* (2nd ed., pp. 122–141). St. Louis, MO: Mosby.

Wilcox, E. M. & Taulli-Lasseigne, J. (2013). Marketing educational activities. In S. L. Bruce (Ed.), *Core curriculum for nursing professional development* (4th ed., pp. 359–374). Chicago: Association for Nursing Professional Development.

Wilkinson, C. S. (2002). Implementing. In B. E. Puetz & J. W. Aucoin (Eds.), *Conversations in nursing professional development* (pp. 157–170). Pensacola, FL: Pohl Publishing.

CHAPTER 11

EVALUATION

BACKGROUND

▶ Evaluation is a systematic, ongoing process, and is based on specific criteria.

▶ Educators, learners, content experts, management, and administration are involved in the evaluation process as appropriate.

▶ Evaluation data are used to revise learning activities to increase their effectiveness and value (American Nurses Association and National Nursing Staff Development Organization, 2010).

▶ The effectiveness of learning activities is directly related to the achievement of learning objectives and impact on job performance.

▶ Methods and levels of evaluation vary from the learner's response to an educational activity through overall program effectiveness. The level selected supports the organization's culture of learning.

▶ The method and level of an evaluation is based on the situation: problem, stakeholders, outcome, data sources, tools available, cost, time, and practicality.

▶ The evaluation data are summarized, documented, and reported, along with outcome achievement, to appropriate persons, including educators, sponsoring agency, clients, and stakeholders (Warren, 2013).

PURPOSES OF EVALUATION

▶ Evaluation is an organized, thorough assessment of educational endeavors. The intellectual process assigns worth, value, and merit to the educational program (Warren, 2013).

▶ It is essential that evaluation be conducted systematically and involve analysis of all activities associated with educational programming.

▶ A goal of evaluation is to improve the effectiveness of educational programs.

▶ The results of evaluation are used to identify future educational needs, appropriate faculty, and effective teaching and learning methodologies.

▶ Evaluation also is conducted to ensure educational programs meet the standards of accrediting organizations.

▶ Evaluation is imperative for the calculation of the benefit–cost ratio of specific learning activities (Avillion, 2005; Warren, 2013, Kirkpatrick, 1998).

TYPES OF EVALUATION

▶ *Competency-based evaluation:* Assessment of a nurse's demonstrated ability to satisfactorily perform specific behaviors essential to the role of the nurse and requirements of the job description, for example, assessment against all competency statements and performance criteria for a specific role during an orientation period.

▶ *Criterion-referenced evaluation:* Evaluation of behaviors in light of specific, predetermined criteria, for example, American Heart Association's Basic Cardiac Life Support course performance checklists for single rescuer and obstructed airway.

▶ *Norm-referenced evaluation:* Evaluation of the achievement of a learner compared to that of other learners, reported as scores or percentages, for example, grading on a curve, the Scholastic Aptitude Test (SAT).

▶ *Formative or process evaluation:* Evaluation of the design process with the purpose of making changes to achieve the goals of the program or to improve outcomes (Fitzpatrick, Sanders, & Worthen, 2004, as cited in Warren, 2013); evaluation can take place during the learning activity and is used to alter content or methods of teaching.

  ▷ Assessment measures for

    ▷ Students: Achievement, satisfaction, teacher observation, written assignments, and small groups

    ▷ Curriculum: Review of syllabi and their delivery, identification of strengths and weaknesses of the curriculum, and classroom observation by a trained observer

▷ Program: Faculty and course program evaluations, cost analysis, participant enrollment and successful completion of the education program (Keating, 2006, p. 551, as cited in Warren, 2013)

▶ *Summative or outcome evaluation:* Evaluation that occurs upon completion of the learning activity and is used to determine final outcomes; provides information to determine program adoption, continuation, or expansion.

▷ Outcome measures (Fitzpatrick et al., 2004, as cited in Warren, 2013):

▷ Link quality of the program to the mission, goals, and objectives of the program.

▷ Quality indicators, performance measures, or patient safety indicators.

▷ Benchmarking used to compare the organization against similar organizations.

METHODOLOGIES OF EVALUATION

Kirkpatrick's Four Levels

▶ *Level 1: Reaction.* The measure of customer satisfaction; sometimes referred to as a "happiness" index. Reaction is essentially the learner's response to the effectiveness of the educator, teaching or learning method, and learning environment, and how well the program was perceived to meet the learning objectives.

▶ *Level 2: Learning.* The extent to which learners acquire knowledge and skills or change attitudes. Learning requires measurement of objective achievement.

▶ *Level 3: Behavior.* The extent to which behavioral changes occur after participating in a learning activity. In addition to presenting an effective education program, other conditions must be met for behavior to change. The learner must want to change, know how and what to do, work in a setting that facilitates the change, and be rewarded for implementing the change.

▶ *Level 4: Results.* The effect the learning activity has on the measures that are important to the organization. Examples of desired results include a decrease in the number of medication errors, decreased staff attrition, an increase in patient satisfaction, or a decrease in the number of nosocomial infections (Kirkpatrick, 1998).

▶ Because many other factors can impact organizational effectiveness, the time and resources devoted to evaluation should relate to the benefits of the evaluation.

▶ Kirkpatrick's model serves as the basis for many evaluation systems.

RSA Model

▶ Developed by Roberta S. Abruzzese for the purpose of conceptualizing evaluations, the RSA model consists of five levels of education and measurement:

1. *Process:* Measures the learner's general satisfaction with the faculty, program content, how well the content met stated objectives, teaching and learning methodologies, and the learning environment.

2. *Content:* Assesses immediate changes in the learner's knowledge, skill, or attitudes after completing a learning activity.

3. *Outcome:* Evaluates changes in the learner's actual nursing practice in the work setting after the completion of a learning activity.

4. *Impact:* Measures organization outcomes that can be attributed, in part, to the effects of a learning experience.

5. *Total Program:* Evaluates the congruence of goals, objectives, accomplishments, and outcomes (Abruzzese, 1996).

CIPP Model

▶ Developed by D. L. Stufflebeam (2003), the CIPP (Context, Input, Process, Product) model examines four aspects of projects and programs for both formative and summative evaluation.

▶ Most notably used for program and system process evaluations

1. *Context:* Assesses data that deal with planning and determining goals, objectives, and priorities.
   Formative: What needs to be done?
   Summative: Were important needs addressed?

2. *Input:* Evaluates internal and external resources, approaches, plans, and goals in relation to feasibility and effectiveness. Data from input evaluation is used for decision-making.
   Formative: How should it be done?
   Summative: Was the effort guided by a defensible plan and budget?

3. *Process:* Assesses implementation of plan (decided from input evaluation) to judge performance and outcomes.
   Formative: Is it being done?
   Summative: Was the service design executed competently and modified as needed?

4. *Product:* Identifies and assesses outcomes in meeting targeted needs.
   Formative: Is it succeeding?
   Summative: Did the effort succeed?

Logic Model

▶ University of Wisconsin Cooperative Extension developed the logic model as a comprehensive framework to be used for program planning, implementation, and evaluation that links investments to results. Components of model include

   ▹ Situation: Problem statement, description, and stakeholders

   ▹ Inputs: Resources invested to achieve the desired outputs

   ▹ Outputs: Lead to the outcomes; outputs consist of the activities, products, or services that reach the targeted participants

   ▹ Outcomes: The changes or benefits for participants, agency, clients; can be short- or long-term; can be positive, negative, or neutral

   ▹ Assumptions: Principles, beliefs, and ideas about the program and participants

   ▹ External factors: The organizational culture, economics, politics, changing priorities, and participant experiences. (University of Wisconsin, 2003, pp. 552–553, as cited in Warren, 2013)

Quality Assurance Model

Donabedian developed a model with 3 parts:

1. *Structure* includes internal and external supports for the program.

2. *Process* is the implementation.

3. *Outcome* measures the quality and extent of program achievement of goals and objectives (Keating, 2006, as cited in Warren, 2013).

Evaluation Instruments

▶ Various tools and resources are required to collect necessary evaluation data.

▶ Examples of tools and resources:

   ▹ Self-rating scales

   ▹ Pre- and posttests

   ▹ Return demonstration in a simulated setting

   ▹ Competency assessment forms

   ▹ Direct observation in the clinical setting

   ▹ Medical record review

   ▹ Review of quality improvement data

- Review of risk management data

- Review of patient, staff, and physician satisfaction surveys

- Organizational performance data

USE OF EVALUATION DATA

The Kirkpatrick (1998) and Abruzzese (1996) models will be used to discuss the use of evaluation data.

Evaluating Reaction and Process Data

▶ It is important to obtain learner reaction regardless of the method of teaching and learning.

▶ The level of learner satisfaction can be correlated to the learner's level of motivation and interest in learning (Kirkpatrick, 1998).

▶ Reaction evaluation data are just as important as other levels of evaluation and should not be discounted; reaction evaluations help to identify effective teaching styles and methods (Avillion, 2005, 2008; Kirkpatrick, 1998).

▶ Data from reaction and process evaluations are reviewed for trends that indicate a need to revise the content, delivery method, or curriculum accordingly.

Evaluating Learning and Content

▶ Positive reactions to a particular learning event are important, but do not indicate actual knowledge acquisition.

▶ Learning is measured by comparing knowledge, skills, or attitudes prior to and after completing an education program.

▶ Start by constructing well-written objectives that measure learning, such as "After completing this self-learning module, the learner accurately calculates pediatric medication doses based on a patient's weight in kilograms 100% of the time."

▶ The type of evaluation is based on the learning domains of the objectives. (See Chapter 3.)

▶ Pretests administered immediately prior to the program give both educators and learners the opportunity to assess current knowledge, and pretests can increase learner motivation.

▶ Note that if a nurse completes a well-written pretest (see "Test Construction" in Chapter 9) successfully, she or he may not need to complete the learning activity.

   ▸ This tactic is especially useful during orientation; pretests can be developed to serve as "challenge" exams.

   ▸ This strategy helps to acknowledge levels of expertise and helps nurses to pursue the education they need, rather than education that is unnecessary or redundant.

▶ Examples of other ways of measuring knowledge acquisition include the use of case studies, group activities, simulations, and demonstration.

▶ The formality of learning and content evaluation is based on the purpose of the learning activity (Avillion, 2005, 2008; Kirkpatrick, 1998).

Evaluating Behavior and Outcome

▶ It is not enough to demonstrate learning as a result of an educational activity.

▶ If learners fail to apply what they have learned, the effectiveness of education is compromised.

▶ Evaluating behavior involves the compilation of data to measure behavioral changes in the clinical setting as a result of participation in a learning activity.

▶ Those who evaluate behavioral change (e.g., peers, managers, educators) must do so consistently.

▶ Evaluators should follow a written set of guidelines that explicitly identify what constitutes appropriate behavioral change.

▶ Results of these evaluations should be shared with the person evaluated, strengths acknowledged, and, if necessary, an action plan for improvement initiated.

▶ The form used to document this type of evaluation should have a place for the signatures of the evaluator and the person evaluated, as well as the results of the evaluation.

▶ If the person being evaluated fails to perform the desired behavior appropriately, the action plan (including objectives and desired date of achievement) should be documented on the evaluation form and signed by both the evaluator and the person being evaluated.

▶ This type of documentation provides a written record of the steps necessary to achieve the objectives.

▶ Ways to evaluate behavior include direct observation, peer review, medical record review, and patient outcomes (Avillion, 2008; Ludeman, 1998).

Evaluating Results or Impact

▶ Evaluation of impact is the process of assessing the results of education that affect organizational functioning.

▶ The data collected when evaluating behavioral change or application of learning form the basis for impact evaluation:

▷ For example, suppose risk management and quality improvement data showed a substantial increase in the occurrence of nosocomial infections, with the causes traced to lack of handwashing, failure to maintain sterile techniques, and failure to initiate antibiotic therapy when the patients' conditions indicated the existence of an infection.

▷ After extensive education offerings were presented to all direct patient care providers, reactions were evaluated and knowledge acquisition was measured by pre- and posttests and case studies.

▷ Behavioral change was assessed by direct observation, medical record audits, and review of patient care plans.

▷ Impact was measured by statistical comparison of the type, number, and cause of nosocomial infections 3 months before and 3 months after the educational offerings.

▷ Improvement was calculated in percentages and evaluated in terms of the total organization, by department, and by unit.

▶ The results of this level of evaluation should be reported to staff, management, and appropriate stakeholders and include data (e.g., infection control, quality improvement, risk management; Avillion, 2005; Shelton & Alliger, 1998).

Measuring Economic Value or Worth

▶ The purpose of evaluating return on investment (ROI) or benefit–cost ratio (BCR) is to measure the effect of education on the financial bottom line.

▶ The assumption is that benefit can be quantified and training is the sole variable in achieving that benefit.

▶ ROI and BCR are not calculated on every learning activity, but only on those that have the most significant impact on organizational effectiveness.

▶ Both measures use annual values because the value of short-term training is most frequently captured within a year (Phillips, 1997).

▶ BCR compares the economic benefit (expressed in dollars) of a program to the cost of the program. The organization establishes an acceptable cost–benefit ratio standard. The formula is:

$$BCR = \frac{\text{Program Benefits}}{\text{Program Costs}}$$

▶ ROI is the program benefits (expressed in dollars) minus the costs of a learning activity. The difference is divided by the costs, then multiplied by 100 so that the ROI is expressed as a percentage:

$$ROI\ (\%) = \frac{(\text{Benefits} - \text{Costs})\ x\ 100}{\text{Costs}}$$

▶ Consider the example in the preceding section concerning the need to decrease the incidence of nosocomial infections. It would be necessary to determine the expenses directly related to the increased rate of nosocomial infections.

  ▸ Expenses include increased length of stay, loss of third-party reimbursement, cost of additional diagnostic procedures and treatments triggered by nosocomial infections, and the cost of any damages paid to the patient or family as a result of malpractice lawsuits related to such infections. Also included are the costs of developing, implementing, and evaluating the learning activities designed to decrease the incidence of nosocomial infections.

  ▸ The benefits include the money saved as a result of decreased length of stay when no nosocomial infections develop, no expenses for additional diagnostic and treatment measures, appropriate third-party reimbursement, and lack of malpractice awards.

▶ ROI demonstrates the financial worth of a learning activity in terms of business and strategic goals. This type of evaluation is complex and takes considerable time and effort.

▶ ROI is "usually recommended for programs with high visibility, are of high importance to administrators, are related to the strategic plan, and have far reaching impact." (DeSilets, 2010, p. 559, as cited by Warren, 2013).

OUTCOME MEASURES

▶ BCR, ROI, and results or impact evaluation are types of outcome measures. However, in health care other performance measures are also considered outcomes measures.

Benchmarking

▶ Benchmarking is the comparison of an organization with one or more organizations or data sets that are considered experts or leaders.

▶ Benchmarking can be performed with a primary competitor, internally among different departments, with organizations of similar size and scope, or with award-winning organizations.

▶ It is an effective means to identify improvements that can make an important difference to an organization.

▶ Benchmarking is done to improve the efficiency or effectiveness of a process to produce the desired outcome. The focus is the process, not the result.

▶ The benchmark is the "ideal" and can be used for a gap analysis, with the educational program designed to bridge that gap.

▶ Program outcome effectiveness is indirectly related to changes against the benchmark.

▶ Examples of benchmark data that can be affected by educational programs are staff vacancy rate, infection rates, employee satisfaction, and quality indicators (Kelly-Thomas, 1998; Marrelli, 1997).

Quality Indicators

▶ Quality indicators (QIs) provide a perspective on the quality of care provided by hospitals.

▶ The Agency for Healthcare Research and Quality (AHRQ) and the Centers for Medicare and Medicaid Services (CMS) set the initial QIs and continue to add to them.

▶ QIs are publicly reported by hospitals.

▶ QIs can assist hospitals in identifying problem areas for further review of processes that affect the outcome measure.

▶ Examples of QIs are mortality rates for stroke and hip replacements, number of hysterectomies, pneumococcal and influenza vaccination status of patients with pneumonia, perioperative urinary catheter removal by postoperative day 2, re-admissions for heart failure, and fall rates (AHRQ, 2006; CMS, 2010).

Performance Measures

▶ The organization selects which measures will become part of its continual performance monitoring.

▶ Tools used for performance monitoring and quality improvement processes include dashboards, scorecards, and report cards.

▶ The purpose of these tools is to keep the performance measures in the forefront of everyday practice.

▶ The sophistication of the tool depends on the resources of the organization. Data can be displayed in traditional charts, graphs, or other indicators such as color-coded grids or gauges.

▶ When process improvements are identified, education or training is most frequently the mechanism employed for correction. However, most process improvements are not corrected by an educational activity. Rather, the educational activity teaches the employee what behavior changes are needed to improve the organization's desired outcome.

▶ Examples of performance measures are quality indicators, national patient safety goals, core measures, and nurse-sensitive indicators.

REFERENCES

Abruzzese, R. S. (Ed.). (1996). *Nursing staff development: Strategies for success.* St. Louis, MO: Mosby.

Agency for Healthcare Research and Quality. (2006). *Inpatient quality indicators overview.* Rockville, MD: Author. Retrieved from http://www.qualityindicators.ahrq.gov/iqi_overview.htm

American Nurses Association and National Nursing Staff Development Organization. (2010). *Nursing professional development: Scope and standards of practice.* Silver Spring, MD: Nursesbooks.org.

Avillion, A. E. (2005). *Nurse educator manual: Essential skills and guidelines for effective practice.* Marblehead, MA: HCPro.

Avillion, A. E. (2008). *A practical guide to staff development: Tools and techniques for effective education* (2nd ed.). Marblehead, MA: HCPro.

Centers for Medicare & Medicaid Services. (2010). *Reporting hospital quality data for annual payment update.* Retrieved from https://www.cms.gov/HospitalQualityInits/08_HospitalRHQDAPU.asp

Donabedian, A. (1996). Evaluating the quality of medical care. *Milbank Memorial Fund Quarterly, 44*(2), 166–206.

Kelly-Thomas, K. J. (1998). *Clinical and nursing staff development: Current competence, future focus* (2nd ed.). Philadelphia: Lippincott.

Kirkpatrick, D. L. (1998). *Evaluating training programs* (2nd ed.). San Francisco: Berrett-Koehler.

Ludeman, K. (1998). Measuring skills and behavior. In D. L. Kirkpatrick, *Another look at evaluating training programs* (pp. 154–158). Alexandria, VA: American Society for Training & Development.

Marelli, T. M. (1997). *The nurse manager's survival guide: Practical answers to everyday problems* (2nd ed.). St. Louis, MO: Mosby.

Phillips, J. J. (1997). *Handbook of training evaluation and measurement methods* (3rd ed.). Oxford, UK: Elsevier.

Shelton, S., & Alliger, G. (1998). Who's afraid of level 4 evaluation? A practical approach. In D. L. Kirkpatrick, *Another look at evaluating training programs* (pp. 171–174). Alexandria, VA: American Society for Training & Development.

Stufflebeam, D. L. (2003). *The CIPP model for evaluation.* Retrieved from http://www.oregoneval.org/program/CIPP%20Model%20for%20Evaluation.pdf

Warren, J. I. (2013). Program evaluation and return on investment. In S. L. Bruce (Ed.), *Core curriculum for nursing professional development* (4th ed., pp. 547–567). Chicago: Association for Nursing Professional Development.

CHAPTER 12

DOCUMENTATION AND RECORDS

BACKGROUND

▶ Documentation is addressed throughout *Nursing Professional Development: Scope and Standards of Practice* (American Nurses Association [ANA] & National Nursing Staff Development Organization [NNSDO], 2010)

   ▷ *Assessment:* "Documents relevant data in a retrievable format" (p. 23)

   ▷ *Identification of Issues and Trends:* "Documents identified needs in a manner that facilitates generation of purpose statements, educational objectives, program content, and evaluation criteria" (p. 24)

   ▷ *Outcomes Identification:* "Documents outcomes, including those that demonstrate learning and program impact" (p. 25)

   ▷ *Planning:* "Documents the planning process" (p. 26)

   ▷ *Implementation:* "Documents implementation and any modifications, including changes or omissions, of the identified plan" (p. 27)

   ▷ *Coordination:* "Documents coordination of the activities" (p. 28)

   ▷ *Evaluation:* "Documents the results of evaluation" (p. 31)

   ▷ *Quality of Nursing Professional Development:* "Documents the evaluation of nursing professional development activities" (p. 32)

   ▷ *Collaboration:* "Documents plans and communications of collaborative endeavors" (p. 36)

> *Ethics:* "Documents that the requirements of the accrediting bodies are consistently followed, reporting relevant issues and information to the respective body" (p. 38)

> *Resource Utilization:* "Documents resource utilization decisions and activities" (p. 41)

RECORD MANAGEMENT

Purposes

▶ Monitor educational programs for their relevance, effectiveness, and efficiency

▶ Comply with established educational standards, accreditation standards, federal and state laws, and licensing regulations

▶ Provide information for ongoing evaluation of the nursing professional development department

▶ Convey information about nursing professional development activities to relevant groups who use information for planning, managing, and decision-making

> External audiences: National accrediting and regulatory agencies, such as The Joint Commission, American Nurses Credentialing Center (ANCC), Occupational Safety and Health Administration (OSHA), state boards of nursing, and state departments of health

> Internal audiences: Administrator of organization, chief nursing officer, nursing professional development unit personnel, education committees (Alspach, 1995)

Types of Records

▶ Documentation records

> Job requirement: Requisites for employment such as license, certificates (e.g., BLS, FHM, ACLS, NRP), occupational health (e.g., vaccinations, titers, TB screening)

> Orientation: Documents for new employees as well as changes in roles, responsibilities, or practice settings within an organization that indicate how competency was assessed and requirement was met

> Ongoing competence: Record of attendance at mandatory training and validation of competency to mitigate risk

> Continuing education: Attendance rosters and evidence of completion of educational activities that further knowledge and skills in profession, role, or practice area

▶ Planning records

  ▸ Educational activity calendar

  ▸ Educational activity files: Records of all elements of an educational activity that can be useful as a record of past activities and a resource for future planning (Johansen, 2009, as cited in Brady-Schluttner, 2013).

▶ Operational records

  ▸ Training and compliance reports of employees' participation in educational activities

  ▸ Distribution lists: Electronic or postal mailing lists

  ▸ Periodic reports: Progress or annual reports that communicate information about projects, educational activities, progress toward goal achievement, or other activities of the nursing professional development department

▶ Resource records

  ▸ Biographical data: Information about the education and experience of planners and presenters that qualifies them for participation in the continuing education process

  ▸ Material resource tracking: Information about use and repair of media and equipment

  ▸ Financial records: Budgets and reports on budget performance (Johansen, 2009, as cited in Brady-Schluttner, 2013)

▶ Market research records

  ▸ Needs assessment findings

  ▸ Educational requests from internal and external audiences (Johansen, 2009, as cited in Brady-Schluttner, 2013).

Maintenance of Records

▶ Educational records can be kept manually or via computer software applications. Have a back-up (hard copy or electronic) so documents are retrievable should there be a natural or unnatural disaster.

▶ Organizations may set policies and guidelines for maintaining records, including how long records need to be kept. Consideration should be given to the requirements of external agencies or accrediting bodies for records retention. For example, The Joint Commission requires retention of orientation and competency records throughout an employee's employment period; the American Nurses Credentialing Center requires that accredited organizations retain continuing nursing education records for 6 years.

▶ Responsibility for educational records may lie with the employee, management, or both.

▶ Educational records may be embedded in a learning management system.

▶ Records may be arranged chronologically, alphabetically, or by activity type, code number, or topic area. Consistency is key in being able to retrieve documents for review and reporting.

▶ Retrieval of documents may be for performance review, accreditation, risk management, and compliance reports for regulatory agencies. Records should include all essential data to be useful when documents are retrieved for any of these purposes.

▶ Access to records is on a need-to-know basis. Confidentiality is guided by organizational human resource and education department policies.

▶ Sophisticated automated systems may include bar-code scanning for employee identification badges, link to time and attendance records, or performance evaluation systems (Kelly-Thomas, 1998; O'Shea, 2002).

ACCREDITATION DOCUMENTATION

▶ Foundational documents for the ANCC accreditation system (ANCC, 2013):

▷ *Nursing Professional Development: Scope and Standards of Practice* (ANA & NNSDO, 2010)

▷ *Code of Ethics for Nurses with Interpretive Statements* (ANA, 2001)

▷ Adult learning principles and behavioral objectives from teaching-learning principles, educational theory, and pedagogical literature (ANCC, 2013).

▶ A provider unit has one or more designated nurse planners responsible for being involved with the entire process of an educational activity and documenting adherence to ANCC Accreditation Program criteria (ANCC, 2013).

▶ Documentation of the following is required for nursing continuing education activities to meet ANCC criteria:

▷ Title and location (if live) of educational activity

▷ Type of activity format: live or enduring

▷ Date live activity presented or, for ongoing enduring activities, date first offered and subsequent review dates

▷ Method and findings of the needs assessment

▷ Description of the target audience

- Names, titles, and expertise of activity planners, presenters, faculty, authors, and content reviewers

- Role held by each Planning Committee member (must include identification of the Nurse Planner and content experts)

- Conflict of interest disclosure statements from planners, presenters, faculty, authors, and content reviewers

- Resolution of conflict of interest for planners, presenters, faculty, authors, and content reviewers, if applicable

- Identified gap in knowledge, skill, or practice for the target audience

- Purpose, objectives, content, and instructional strategies of the activity

- Evidence of learner feedback mechanisms

- Method or process used to verify participation of learners

- Rationale and criteria for judging successful completion

- Marketing and promotional material

- Evidence of accreditation or approval statement provided to learners prior to start of educational activity

- Evidence of disclosing to learners the purpose, objectives, criteria for successful completion, presence or absence of conflicts of interest, sponsorship or commercial support, and expiration date of enduring materials

- Means of ensuring content integrity in the presence of commercial support or sponsorship (if applicable)

- Coprovider, sponsorship and commercial support agreements with signatures and dates (if applicable)

- Template of evaluation tool and summative evaluation

- Number of contact hours awarded, including method of calculation

- Documentation of completion with title and date of activity, name and address of provider, number of contact hours, accreditation or approval statement, and participant name

- Participant names and addresses with unique identifiers (ANCC, 2013)

▶ ANCC (2013) requires records be kept in a secure and confidential manner for a period of 6 years.

REFERENCES

Alspach, J. G. (1995). *The educational process in nursing staff development.* St. Louis, MO: Mosby.

American Nurses Association. (2001). *Code of ethics for nurses with interpretive statements.* Washington, DC: American Nurses Publishing.

American Nurses Association and National Nursing Staff Development Organization. (2010). *Nursing professional development: Scope and standards of practice.* Silver Spring, MD: Nursesbooks.org.

American Nurses Credentialing Center. (2013). *2013 ANCC primary accreditation application manual for providers and approvers.* Silver Spring, MD: Author.

Brady-Schluttner, K. (2013). Record keeping. In S. L. Bruce (Ed.), *Core curriculum for nursing professional development* (4th ed., pp. 453–469). Chicago: Association for Nursing Professional Development.

Kelly-Thomas, K. J. (1998). *Clinical and nursing staff development: Current competence, future focus* (2nd ed.). Philadelphia: Lippincott.

O'Shea, K. L. (2002). *Staff development nursing secrets.* Philadelphia: Hanley & Belfus, Inc.

CHAPTER 13

COMMUNICATION

BACKGROUND

▶ *In Nursing Professional Development: Scope and Standards of Practice* (American Nurses Association [ANA] & National Nursing Staff Development Organization [NNSDO], 2010), Standard 10, *Collegiality*, requires the nursing professional development (NPD) specialist to interact with peers, students, colleagues, and others, to share knowledge and skills, and provide constructive feedback to peers regarding their practice. These activities require communication skills.

Follow ANA's *Principles for Social Networking and the Nurse* (ANA, 2011).

Listening Skills

▶ Realize that listening is an active process that requires skill, discipline, and practice.

▶ Concentrate on the words and behavior of the speaker without passing judgment.

▶ Be supportive of self-expression.

▶ Be aware that the goal of listening is to understand.

▶ Listen with genuine interest.

▶ Minimize distractions.

▶ Establish and maintain eye contact, giving full attention to the speaker.

▶ Paraphrase as needed to clarify.

▶ NEVER interrupt.

▶ Pay attention to nonverbal communication (Harvey & Sims, 2003).

Communication Tips

▶ Watch language; avoid technical terms and acronyms that might not be understood by all.

▶ Use fewer words.

▶ Ask open ended questions.

▶ Respect each other's viewpoints and opinions.

▶ Use body language to show interest.

▶ Get feedback from staff members.

▶ Use communication to build "USA": understanding, support, and acceptance.

▶ Communicate purpose and listen without prejudice (Harvey & Sims, 2003; LaBarre, 2004).

▶ Conduct communication at the proper time and place.

Potential Barriers to Effective Communication

▶ Misperceptions: Information received not as intended by speaker

▶ Misinterpretations: Not all information received or distorted by receiver

▶ Faulty reasoning: Information received does not make sense or disparity with visual message

▶ Selective perception: Information received is filtered through fears and barriers

▶ False assumptions: Unspoken assumptions affect trust

▶ Status: Differences in power or status interfere

▶ Gender differences: Style, terms, detail, personal content differences

▶ Cultural differences: Patterns of behavior, beliefs, and values differ from each other (Lovlien, 2013)

NEGOTIATION SKILLS

▶ Definitions

    ▹ *Networking:* "Aligning oneself with others to obtain information, ideas, advice, power, and influence" (Zimmerman & Jones, 2002, p. 167)

    ▹ *Consensus-building:* Pre–decision-making process of informal meetings, discussion, and agreements on issues on a personal level; an effective form of negotiation

    ▹ *Negotiation:* Dialogue process in which two or more parties compromise to reach agreement on course of action to meet synergistic goals and objectives

▶ Negotiation requires input and compromise from stakeholders.

▶ The most effective negotiation process has a win-win outcome (Zimmerman & Jones, 2002).

Development of Trust in Negotiation

▶ Research and prepare beforehand

▶ Observe for behavior reflecting dishonesty

▶ Maintain and share notes

▶ Develop plans

▶ Demonstrate respect (Thurman, 2013)

Negotiating Strategies With Various Types of People

▶ *Adversaries*—low agreement and low trust

    ▹ State the vision of the project.

    ▹ State in a neutral way your own best understanding of the adversary's position.

    ▹ Identify your own contributions to the problem.

    ▹ End the meeting with your own plans and no demand.

▶ *Opponents*—low agreement and high trust

    ▹ Reaffirm the quality of the relationship and mutual trust.

    ▹ State your own position.

    ▹ State in a neutral way what you believe to be the opponent's position.

    ▹ Problem-solve.

▶ *Allies*—high agreement and high trust

 » Affirm agreement.

 » Reaffirm the quality of the trusting relationship.

 » Acknowledge doubts and vulnerabilities related to the project.

 » Ask for advice and support.

▶ *Bedfellows*—high agreement and low trust

 » Reaffirm the agreement.

 » Acknowledge caution.

 » Be clear about what one wants from the bedfellow.

 » Ask what the bedfellow wants and expects.

 » Try to agree about how to work together (Marriner-Tomey, 2004).

Crucial Conversations

▶ Method described by Patternson, Grenny, McMillan and Switzler (2002, as cited in Lovlien, 2013, p. 813) includes

 » Identification of reason for discussion

 » Creation of mutual respect and purpose

 » Use of clarifying statement about what is wanted and not wanted

 » Maintenance of individual safety

 » Commitment to find the common purpose

 » Share facts, story, seek input, ask questions

 » Hear other story, agree on action

 » Identify actions and who will do what

Team-Building

▶ "Team building is an intentional process" (Chitty & Black, 2010, p. 219).

▶ The nursing professional development specialist models team-building behaviors: shows respect to others, builds trust, identifies problematic feelings and misperceptions and corrects them, involves team members in decision-making, and promotes a caring and supportive practice (Chitty & Black, 2010).

Characteristics of Cultures That Support Teams

▶ Value employees' need for relationships with others.

▶ Promote cooperative rather than competitive relationships.

▶ Encourage individual accountability and responsibility.

▶ Recognize individual contributions.

▶ Have positive visions of the future.

▶ Have short- and long-term goals.

▶ Have quality standards.

▶ Believe in their products and services.

▶ Are people-oriented.

▶ Support the community (Marriner-Tomey, 2004).

Group Development

▶ Phases are inevitable and necessary for teams to grow, solve problems, and produce results.

▶ Teams may revert to earlier stages in response to changing circumstances such as change in leadership.

  ▹ *Forming:* The first stage of team-building; the task is one of orientation; members are dependent on the leader

  ▹ *Storming:* Different ideas compete for consideration; emotional response to task demands; members resist group influence

  ▹ *Norming:* Trust begins and motivation increases; open exchange of personal opinions; cohesiveness develops

  ▹ *Performing:* Constructive action; group energy is focused on the task; group interpersonal structure is functional

  ▹ *Adjourning:* Mourning; completion of task with group disengaging; may lead to transformational synergy in performance (Tuckman, 2001)

Skills Needed by Teams

▶ Honesty (articulate current reality openly; identify what is really happening versus what members wish were happening)

▶ Ability to organize and run effective meetings by assigning roles, establishing ground rules for conduct, setting procedures to follow, and following a written agenda

▶ Using team-building activities such as courtesy, improving communication, becoming better able to perform everyday work tasks together, and building strong relationships to develop cohesiveness

▶ Creating an environment that promotes learning, which leads to a shared understanding and effective problem-solving (Gloe, 1998)

Benefits of Self-Managed Teams

▶ Increased productivity

▶ Commitment to the organization and to the job

▶ Common commitment to goals and values

▶ Shared ownership and responsibility for tasks

▶ Proactive approach to problems

▶ Faster response to change

▶ Flexible work practices

▶ Motivation through peer pressure rather than management mandates

▶ Increased employee satisfaction

▶ Better work climate (Marriner-Tomey, 2004)

Professional and Social Networking

▶ Online social networking

  ▷ Social networking sites are websites where you can share information and communicate with other people. These sites usually used in the form of a personal profile, elements of which other people can see.

  ▷ This technology enables members to keep in touch with their friends and acquaintances.

  ▷ Social networks also focus on building online communities among people who share similar interests or activities.

  ▷ Online social networking offers the ability to connect with friends, chat, and organize social events. These websites (e.g., Facebook, LinkedIn, Google+, Twitter) have made certain aspects of life easier and are powerful tools for communication, but have also blurred the line between personal and professional lives.

▹ Nurses need to be aware of the requirements of the Health Insurance Portability and Accountability Act (HIPAA) to ensure that they do not post patient information or photos to social networks. Improper use of social network sites can result in personal liability for defamation, invasion of privacy, or harassment.

▶ Risks of social networking

▹ Connecting to unknown persons or people who act unprofessionally

▹ Risk of identity theft

▹ Posting behavior or pictures that are not professional. These may result in disciplinary actions, up to and including termination.

▹ Combining friends, coworkers, and acquaintances into a single venue risks blending the personal and professional environments. The information you post may be on view to current or potential employers, patients, and professional colleagues.

▹ Professional reputation can be negatively affected by information available online.

▹ "Members only" discussions (e.g., private email groups) may show your professional email signature that can identify your facility, situation, or other information that unwittingly violates hospital policies (Stokowski, 2011).

▹ Information can take on a life of its own when inaccuracies become "fact" (ANA, 2011).

▶ Boards of Nursing may investigate inappropriate disclosures on the grounds of

▹ Unprofessional conduct

▹ Unethical conduct

▹ Moral turpitude

▹ Mismanagement of patient records

▹ Revealing privilege communications

▹ Breach of conduct (National Council of State Boards of Nursing [NCSBN], 2011)

▶ Advantages of social networking

▹ Instant dissemination of knowledge to offer just-in-time training

▹ Forum for collegial interchange

▹ Ability to discuss and debate issues pertinent to education, practice, and research at a global level

▹ Enables professional connections and mentoring relationships

- Ability to participate in discussions regardless of geographic location or time zone

- Opportunity to network with other professionals and nurture these relationships

- Opportunity to educate the public on nursing and health-related matters

▶ General guidelines for social networking

- Make your profile private and monitor who can see your information.

- Allow only known friends or acquaintances to view your information.

- Use discretion and common sense when posting a status or photo that is public.

- Post comments or photos during off-work hours.

- Follow your institution's social media policy, developed by the institution to protect itself from the online actions of employees or students.

  ▷ The social media policy should be a component of orientation and identified in educational programs as warranted.

- Follow NCSBN's guidelines for social media

  ▷ Nurses have an ethical and legal obligation to maintain patient privacy and confidentiality at all times.

  ▷ Do not transmit any patient-related images or information on electronic media.

  ▷ Do not identify any patient or family information.

  ▷ Do not refer to patients in a disparaging or descriptive manner, even if their identity is not identified.

  ▷ Do not take photos or videos of patients using personal devices, including cell phones or tablet devices.

  ▷ Maintain professional boundaries while posting to electronic media. Just like in face-to-face interaction, the nurse has the responsibility to enforce professional boundaries with the patient in the online environment.

COLLABORATION

Definition

▶ Collaboration is not just cooperation, but the concerted effort of individuals and groups to achieve a shared goal.

▶ "The NPD specialist collaborates with the interprofessional teams, leaders, stakeholders, and others to facilitate nursing practice and positive outcomes for consumers" (ANA & NNSDO, 2010, p. 36).

Strategies for Successful Collaboration

▶ Develop collegial relationships with managers to identify staff learning needs and assure management follow-up.

▶ Learn to relate to nursing staff in a nonthreatening, supportive manner.

▶ Develop close rapport with nursing staff.

▶ Find out what motivates staff members to improve their performance so leaders can awaken their motivation.

▶ Listen carefully to the messages received from managers, staff members, and colleagues; clarify and validate them (Lewis & Case, 2001).

▶ Collaboration for positive outcomes in nursing practice include

▷ Engagement of key interprofessional stakeholders

▷ Partnerships with internal and external parties

▷ Education, programs, and consultation

▷ Creation of life-long learning opportunities

▷ Measurement of outcomes (Thurman, 2013, p. 833)

FEEDBACK

▶ Definition: "Specific knowledge given to participants of learning results" (Ellis & O'Connell, 2009, p. 60).

▶ Feedback is a critical requirement of sustained high-level performance.

▶ A lack of feedback leads to unsatisfactory performance.

▶ Specific, frequent feedback is the quickest, cheapest, and most effective intervention for improving performance.

Characteristics of Feedback

▶ Starts with clear expectations

▶ Specific, not general (for example, "Your documentation was clear, thorough, and concise" rather than "Your documentation was good")

▶ Given as close to the event as possible

▶ Content addresses correct performance

▶ Focus is on behavior, not the person

▶ Provided sincerely and honestly with an intent to help

▶ Shares information and observations, not advice

▶ Feedback discussion begins with a specific statement of the problem with expected performance.

▶ Focuses on "next time" rather than looking backward

Types of Feedback

▶ *Negative* feedback consists of put-downs, is not useful, and is typically nonspecific.

▶ *Neutral* feedback is a statement of a problem with no direction toward improvement.

▶ *Positive* feedback is a specific statement of what and how performance was done well.

▶ *Constructive* feedback provides direction for how to improve performance.

▶ *Recognition* feedback (i.e., a job well done) is a powerful motivator (Fournies, 2000; Peters, 2000).

POSITIVISM

Appreciative Inquiry

▶ Look for what works in an organization.

▶ Construct statements of what could be, based on what has been.

▶ Collective strengths can transform an organization.

▶ Memories of positive occurrences create a positive atmosphere within the organization.

▶ The 4 phases of inquiry are

1. *Discovery:* Search to understand the best of what is and has been

2. *Dream:* Engage in thinking big, out of the box

3. *Design:* Make choices for transformation

4. *Destiny:* Focus on personal and organizational commitments (Cooperrider & Whitney, 2005)

▶ Examples of appreciative questions:

▹ What do you love the most about being a preceptor? (Discovery)

▹ What would make for better patient safety? (Dream)

▹ In what areas do you most affect patient care? (Design)

▹ How would you personally like to be involved in the unit's self-governance? (Destiny)

CONFLICT MANAGEMENT

General Information on Conflict

▶ Conflict is as inevitable as change.

▶ Conflict is not always negative; it can be a powerful impetus for positive change.

▶ Conflicts result from a disparity between real or perceived goals, values, roles, attitudes, or actions of two or more persons or groups.

▶ Conflict may be individual (within one person), interpersonal (between two or more persons), intragroup (within a group), or intergroup (between two or more groups).

▶ Managing conflict is highly individualized, but skills in this area are critical for nurses (Grant & Massey, 1999).

Framework for Conflict Assessment

PEPRS framework

▶ *Persons:* Identify all involved parties, including their perceptions of the conflict, gender, socioeconomic background, cultural background, and professional socialization.

▶ *Events and issues:* Develop a clear picture of the triggering events; the surrounding historical context; the level of interdependence among the participants; the issues, goals, and resources; and previously considered solutions.

▶ *Power:* Assess the impact of power on the conflict; all conflicts are based on attempts to protect participants' self-esteem or change perceived inequities in power because most participants believe that the other person or persons have the greater power in the situation.

▶ *Regulation:* Resources potentially available to regulate the conflict, including internal and external factors, previous resolution attempts, or a neutral third party

▶ *Style:* Be cognizant of the influence of the conflict management style used (Sportsman, 2005).

Modes of Conflict Management

▶ The Thomas-Kilmann Conflict Mode Instrument looks at two dimensions of behavior: assertiveness ("extent to which the person attempts to satisfy his own concerns") and cooperativeness ("extent to which the person attempts to satisfy the other person's concerns").

▶ These two dimensions define five different modes of response to conflict:

1. *Competing:* Assertive and uncooperative; pursues own concerns at the other person's expense

2. *Accommodating:* Unassertive and cooperative; neglects own concerns to satisfy others' concerns; complete opposite of competing mode

3. *Avoiding:* Unassertive and uncooperative; pursues neither ones own or others' concerns

4. *Collaborating:* Assertive and cooperative; works with others to satisfy their concerns; complete opposite of avoiding

5. *Compromising:* Moderately assertive and moderately cooperative; finds mutually acceptable solution to both parties' concerns

▶ We are capable of all five modes, but typically rely on the modes with which we are most adept based on temperament or practice (Thomas & Kilmann, 2007).

REFERENCES

American Nurses Association. (2001). *Code of ethics for nurses with interpretive statements.* Washington, DC: American Nurses Publishing.

American Nurses Association. (2011). *Principles for social networking and the nurse.* Silver Spring, MD: Author

American Nurses Association and National Nursing Staff Development Organization (2010). *Nursing professional development: Scope and standards of practice.* Silver Spring, MD: Nursesbooks.org.

Chitty, K. K., & Black, B. P. (2010). *Professional nursing: Concepts and challenges* (6th ed.). Maryland Heights, MD: Saunders Elsevier.

Cooperrider, D. L., & Whitney, D. (2005). *Appreciative inquiry: A positive revolution in change.* San Francisco: Berrett-Koehler Publishers.

Ellis, N. F., & O'Connell, K. M. (2009). Principles of adult learning. In S. L. Bruce (Ed.), *Core curriculum for staff development* (3rd ed., pp. 33–65). Pensacola, FL: National Nursing Staff Development Organization.

Fournies, F. F. (2000). *Coaching for improved work performance* (rev. ed.). New York: McGraw-Hill.

Gloe, D. (1998). Quality management: A staff development tradition. In K. J. Kelley-Thomas (Ed.), *Clinical and nursing staff development: Current competence, future focus* (2nd ed., pp. 301–336). Philadelphia: Lippincott-Raven.

Grant, A. B., & Massey, V. H. (1999). *Nursing leadership, management, and research.* Springhouse, PA: Springhouse.

Harvey, E., & Sims, P. (2003). *Nuts'n bolts leadership: "How to" strategies and practical tips for leaders at ALL levels.* Dallas: Walk the Talk.

LaBarre, P. (2004). The agenda—grassroots leadership. In G. M. Spreitzer & K. H. Perttula (Eds.), *Wiley/Fast Company reader series: Leadership* (pp. 49–56). Hoboken, NJ: Wiley.

Lewis, D. J., & Case, B. (2001). The staff development specialist role. In A. E. Avillion (Ed.), *Core curriculum for staff development* (2nd ed., pp. 91–105). Pensacola, FL: National Nursing Staff Development Organization.

Lovlien, C. (2013). Elements of nursing professional development practice: Leader/communicator. In S. L. Bruce (Ed.), *Core curriculum for nursing professional development* (4th ed., pp. 799–826). Chicago: Association for Nursing Professional Development.

Marriner-Tomey, A. (2004). *Guide to nursing management and leadership* (7th ed.). St Louis, MO: Mosby-Year Book.

National Council of State Boards of Nursing. (2011). *White paper: A nurse's guide to the use of social media.* Retrieved from https://www.ncsbn.org/Social_Media.pdf

Peters, P. (2000). *Seven tips for delivering performance feedback.* Retrieved from http://www.performance-appraisals.org/cgi-bin/links/jump.cgi?ID=10434

Sportsman, S. (2005). Build a framework for conflict assessment. *Nursing Management, 36*(4), 32, 34–36, 38, 40.

Stokowski, L. A. (2011). *Social media and nurses: Promising or perilous?* Retrieved from http://www.medscape.com/viewarticle/753317

Thomas, K. W., & Kilmann, R. H. (2007). *Conflict and conflict management.* Retrieved from http://www.kilmann.com/conflict.html

Thurman, S. (2013). Elements of nursing professional development practice: Collaboration/advisor/mentor. In S. L. Bruce (Ed.), *Core curriculum for nursing professional development* (4th ed., pp. 829–846). Chicago: Association for Nursing Professional Development.

Tuckman, B. W. (2001). Developmental sequence in small groups. *Group Facilitation: A Research and Applications Journal, 3,* 66–80.

Zimmerman, P. G., & Jones, C. L. (2002). Negotiation. In P. G. Zimmerman (Ed.), *Nursing management secrets* (pp. 167–170). Philadelphia: Hanley & Belfus.

CHAPTER 14

CURRENT THEORIES OF CHANGE MANAGEMENT

BACKGROUND

▶ The nursing professional development (NPD) specialist serves as a change facilitator by analyzing the need for change; incorporating changes into educational activities; and using collaboration, facilitation, and problem-solving skills to support the change process. The NPD specialist "exhibits creativity and flexibility through times of change" (American Nurses Association [ANA] & National Nursing Staff Development Organization [NNSDO], 2010, p. 42).

▶ Change is the process of altering or replacing existing knowledge, skills, attitudes, systems, policies, or procedures.

▶ Though change is a dynamic process that necessitates alterations in behavior and usually causes some conflict and resistance, it can also stimulate positive behaviors and attitudes and improve organizational outcomes and employee performance.

▶ Change can be the result of identified problems in existing knowledge, skills, and systems, or of the need to change established ways of conducting business because of alterations in knowledge, technology, management, or leadership.

▶ Problems are identified from many sources, including risk management data, quality improvement data, employee performance evaluations, and accreditation survey results.

▶ The Institute of Medicine (IOM) *Crossing the Quality Chasm* report in 2001 called for major healthcare reform and the *Future of Nursing* report in 2011 called for the expansion of nursing practice and the increase of baccalaureate-prepared RNs.

▶ Change may be necessary due to changes in organizational structure or goals; accreditation criteria; economic drivers; or advances in diagnosis, treatment, and patient outcomes.

▶ Change at any level requires different behavior from the people involved.

▶ Skills needed to effect change include leadership, management, political savvy, analytical, interpersonal, system, business, and communication skills (Nickols, 2007; O'Shea, 2002).

▶ Systems change demands a "drastic shift in locus of control, accountability, expectations, performance, and measurement" (Malloch & Porter-O'Grady, 2006).

▶ The outcomes of change must be consistent with organizational mission, vision, and values.

▶ Because change is a constant in the healthcare environment, it is important to remember key points:

  ▹ Employees will react differently to change, no matter how important or advantageous the change is purported to be.

  ▹ Basic needs will influence reaction to change, such as the need to be part of the change process, the need to be able to express oneself openly and honestly, and the need to feel that one has some control over the impact of change.

  ▹ Change often results in loss (e.g., downsizing, changes in established routines) and employees may react with shock, anger, and resistance, and, hopefully, ultimate acceptance.

  ▹ Change must be managed realistically, without false hopes and expectations, yet with enthusiasm for the future.

  ▹ It is important that management deal with the fears and concerns triggered by change in an honest manner (Monaghan, 2009; Team Technology, 2014).

CHANGE THEORIES

▶ Below is a sample of both classic and current change theories. This list is not meant to be all-inclusive.

▶ Lewin's Change Theory

▷ A three-step model based on the premise that behavior is a dynamic balance of forces working in opposition. Driving forces facilitate change by pushing employees in a desired direction, and inhibiting forces hamper change because they push employees in the opposite direction.

▷ Step 1 is the process of altering behavior to "unfreeze," or agitate the status quo (equilibrium state). Step 1 is necessary if resistance is to be overcome and conformity achieved.

▷ Step 2, "change," involves movement of the employees to a new level of equilibrium. It helps employees view change from a new perspective, work together to achieve desired outcomes of change, and facilitate consistency among management and employees.

▷ Step 3 is "refreezing," or attaining equilibrium with the newly desired behaviors. Step 3 occurs after change is implemented so that new behaviors and desired outcomes can be integrated into the organization (Lewin, 1951).

▶ Lippitt's Seven-Step Change Theory

▷ Expands Lewin's theory to place additional emphasis on the role of the change agent.

▷ Step 1: Diagnose the problem by examining all possible consequences, determining who will be affected by the change, identifying essential management personnel who will be responsible for fixing the problem, collecting data from those who will be affected by the change, and ensuring that those affected by the change will be committed to its success.

▷ Step 2: Evaluate motivation and capability for change by identifying financial and human resources capacity and organizational structure.

▷ Step 3: Assess the change agent's motivation and resources, experience, stamina, and dedication.

▷ Step 4: Select progressive change objectives by defining the change process and developing action plans and accompanying strategies.

▷ Step 5: Explain the role of the change agent to all involved employees (e.g., expert, facilitator, consultant) and ensure that expectations are clear.

▷ Step 6: Maintain change by facilitating feedback, enhancing communication, and coordinating the effects of change.

▷ Step 7: Gradually terminate the helping relationship of the change agent (Lippitt, Watson, & Wesley, 1958).

▶ Rogers' Five-Stage Change Theory

» Stage 1: Impart knowledge in terms of the reason for the change, how it will occur, and who will be involved.

» Stage 2: Persuade employees to accept change by relaying essential information and note that attitudes, both favorable and unfavorable, are formed.

» Stage 3: Decide whether to ultimately adopt the change by analyzing data and implementing a pilot study or trial of the new processes triggered by the change.

» Stage 4: Implement the change on a more permanent or established basis as the organization evolves to accommodate the change.

» Stage 5: Confirm adoption of the change by the employees responsible for and affected by the change (Rogers & Shoemaker, 1971).

▶ Transitions Theory

» "Model for analyzing the human behavioral response to predictable and unpredictable change" (Meleis, 2010, p. 754, as cited in Berry, 2013)

▹ Characteristics include process with beginning and end, disconnectedness, perception, and patterns of response.

▹ Categories of transitions

▷ Developmental

▷ Situational

▷ Health–illness

▷ Organizational

▶ Appreciative Inquiry

» Appreciative inquiry (AI) takes an opposite approach. Rather than define a problem, AI looks at what works in an organization. Positive questions are asked to see potentials and possibilities to move toward.

» There are four stages to the cycle of AI:

1. Discovery: Asking relevant stakeholders what is already positive in current practice: what is.

2. Dream: Through the use of imagination, create a clear vision for the future: what might be.

3. Design: Based on positive past achievements, identify the positive actions needed to reach the "dream": how to get there.

4. Destiny: Creating a climate for positive sustainable change: positive empowerment.

▹ Central to AI's theory are five underlying principles:

1. Constructionist Principle: People create their reality by how they view the world (organization).

2. Poetic Principle: Organizations, like poems, are open to infinite interpretation.

3. Simultaneity Principle: Change occurs as we talk about it.

4. Anticipatory Principle: Change is what we view as our future.

5. Positive Principle: Positive questions lead to positive images, which lead to positive energy and relationships (Cooperrider & Whitney, 2001).

MANAGEMENT OF CHANGE: BASIC CONCEPTS

▶ Change management is the process of making changes in a deliberate, planned, and systematic manner.

▶ Change management uses theories, models, methods and techniques, tools, and skills.

▶ Knowledge of change management is drawn from numerous disciplines (e.g., psychology, business management, economics, engineering, organizational behavior).

▶ The goal of change management is to implement change efficiently for the benefit of the organization.

▶ Change has both content and process dimensions. Addressing underlying processes and effective communication of the change expectations leads to a successful change initiative.

▶ At the core of effective change are clearly defined outcomes of the proposed change, identified actions to attain the outcomes, and implementation of those actions (Monaghan, 2009; Nickols, 2007).

Creating a Climate for Effective Change

▶ Recognize that change is never easy and will be met with enthusiasm by some and resistance by others.

▶ Identify those who will be enthusiastic about the change (early adopters) and those who will be resistors (laggers); involve them to build momentum and identify barriers, respectively.

▶ Collect and analyze data so that the need for change (and its consequences) can be clearly articulated.

▶ Give employees information honestly and allow them to ask questions and express concerns.

▶ Articulate the reasons for change, how it will affect employees, how it will benefit the organization, and the desired outcomes of the change process.

▶ Ensure leadership commitment so that leaders, in turn, can provide consistent information to staff members (Jones, Aquirre, & Calderone, 2004; Monaghan, 2009; Nickols, 2007).

Resistance to Change

▶ Anticipate barriers to change, including components of organizational structure, and take action to remove them. Diffuse power groups and processes to prevent large barriers from systems and stakeholders (Porter-O'Grady & Malloch, 2003).

▶ Employees are resistant to change for a variety of reasons:

  ▹ Fear of losing one's job, having to acquire new skills, and losing the ability to work effectively in a changed environment

  ▹ Fear of losing one's unofficial power or influence

  ▹ Failure to understand the reasons for change

  ▹ Failure to understand how the change will benefit the workplace

  ▹ Failure of management to involve affected employees in the change process

  ▹ Failure of management to communicate effectively (e.g., not providing the reason for or full breadth of the change, limiting information to a few individuals, limiting methods used for communication)

  ▹ Failure of management to relay facts about the change process honestly and realistically (Monaghan, 2009; Nickols, 2007)

▶ Change resistors must be identified, worked with, challenged, and placed in the midst of the change process so as not to impede the change (Porter-O'Grady & Malloch, 2003).

The Process of Managing Change

- ▶ Assessment phase
  - ▹ Identify problem or opportunity for change
  - ▹ Collect and analyze data
  - ▹ Recognize driving and restraining forces
  - ▹ Identify potential for resistance
- ▶ Planning (unfreezing) phase
  - ▹ Know the target system for the change
  - ▹ Assemble a team
  - ▹ Create a process and operational indicators
  - ▹ Establish a timeline for feedback and evaluation of progress
- ▶ Implementation phase
  - ▹ Initiate plans
  - ▹ Create a supportive environment
  - ▹ Provide information
  - ▹ Provide training
  - ▹ Select key stakeholders to support the change
  - ▹ Value participants' input
  - ▹ Ensure team has appropriate authority to act
- ▶ Recognize and address conflicts
  - ▹ Reward desired behaviors
- ▶ Evaluation (refreezing) phase
  - ▹ Monitor operational indicators
  - ▹ Evaluate effectiveness
  - ▹ Stabilize the change (Mick, 2011, as cited in Berry, 2013)

REFERENCES

American Nurses Association and National Nursing Staff Development Organization. (2010). *Nursing professional development: Scope and standards of practice.* Silver Spring, MD: nursesbooks.org.

Berry, M. (2013). Change agent/team member. In S. L. Bruce (Ed.), *Core curriculum for nursing professional development* (4th ed., pp. 751–777). Chicago: Association for Nursing Professional Development.

Cooperrider, D. L., & Whitney, D. (2001). A positive revolution in change: Appreciative inquiry. Retrieved from http://appreciativeinquiry.case.edu/uploads/whatisai.pdf

Jones, J., Aquirre, D., & Calderone, M. (2004). 10 principles of change management. *Strategy+Business.* Retrieved from http://www.strategy-business.com/article/rr00006?pg=all

Institute of Medicine. (2001). *Crossing the quality chasm: A new health system for the 21st century.* Washington DC: The National Academies Press. Retrieved from http:www.iom.edu/Reports/2001/Crossing-the-Quality-Chasm-A-New-HealthSystem-for-the-21st-Century.aspx

Institute of Medicine. (2011). *The future of nursing: Leading change, advancing health.* Washington, DC: The National Academies Press. Retrieved from http://iom.edu/Reports/2010/The-Future-of-Nursing-Leading-Change-Advancing-Health.aspx

Lewin, K. (1951). *Field theory in social science.* New York: Harper & Row.

Lippitt, R., Watson, J., & Westley, B. (1958). *The dynamics of planned change.* New York: Harcourt, Brace & World.

Malloch, K., & Porter-O'Grady, T. (2006). *Introduction to evidence-based practice in nursing and health care.* Sudbury, MA: Jones & Bartlett.

Monaghan, H. M. (2009). Change & change agents. In S. L. Bruce (Ed.), *Core curriculum for staff development* (3rd ed., pp. 111–137). Pensacola, FL: National Nursing Staff Development Organization.

Nickols, F. (2007). *Change management 101: A primer.* Retrieved from http://www.nickols.us/change.pdf

O'Shea, K. L. (2002). *Staff development nursing secrets.* Philadelphia: Hanley & Belfus.

Porter-O'Grady, T., & Malloch, K. (2003). *Quantum leadership: A textbook of new leadership.* Sudbury, MA: Jones & Bartlett.

Rogers, E., & Shoemaker, F. (1971). *Communication of innovations: A cross-cultural approach.* New York: Free Press.

Team Technology. (2014). Change management: Five basic principles, and how to apply them. *Team Technology.* Retrieved from http://www.teamtechnology.co.uk/changemanagement.html

CHAPTER 15

RESOURCE MANAGEMENT

BACKGROUND

▶ The American Nurses Association's (American Nurses Association [ANA] & National Nursing Staff Development Organization [NNSDO], 2010) Standard 15, **Resource Utilization**, states "the nursing professional development specialist considers factors related to safety, effectiveness, and cost in regard to professional development activities and expected outcomes" (p. 41).

TEAM MANAGEMENT

▶ See Chapter 13 section on team-building for further information.

▶ Regular feedback to teams is important for performance and to identify where the team fits into the "big picture."

▶ Clearly identify expectations and goals.

▶ Delegate tasks based on competency of the team member, complexity of the task, and potential outcome.

▶ Address conflicts as they arise; the longer a problem is allowed to fester within a team, the more energy and emotion it will take to solve.

▶ Have the courage to accept responsibility, seek the truth, take risks, and stand up for what's right.

▶ Give the team the freedom to be successful.

▶ Give feedback on performance.

▶ Establish strategies to promote recognition of nursing professional development (NPD) specialists personally and within the organization.

PROJECT MANAGEMENT

▶ See Chapter 16, Project Management.

FISCAL MANAGEMENT

▶ *Standards of Professional Performance for Nursing Professional Development*, Standard 15 (quoted at beginning of chapter) states the NPD specialist:

> "[A]llocates human, financial, and material resources based on identified needs and goals
>
> Develops innovative solutions and strategies to secure appropriate resources and technology for professional development activities" (ANA & NNSDO, 2010, p. 41).

▶ See Chapter 10 of this book for definitions of budgeting terms.

▶ Budgets can be defined by scope (e.g., project budget, department budget), purpose (e.g., supply budget, personnel budget), and time frame (e.g., monthly budget, annual budget; Smith, 2002).

▶ Determine department budget.

- Look at past expenditures and revenue to assist with operating and capital budgets.

- Operating budget: Used to account for revenue and expenses of day-to-day operations; includes income from and costs of goods and services, personnel costs, supplies, and equipment.

- Capital budget: Long-range planning for major cost items such as physical changes, major equipment and inventories, and depreciation costs.

▶ Monitor budget.

- Compare projected versus actual costs (variances) on a regular basis.

- Document variances, both anticipated and unanticipated.

- Implement cost-containment and reduction strategies as needed to keep costs within acceptable limits for volume.

- Ensure all personnel are aware of costs (Avillion, Brunt, & Ferrell, 2007).

▶ Uses for a budget

    » Document fiscal accountability of the professional development unit.

    » Identify and monitor trends in use of resources.

    » Evaluate educational activities and departmental functions from a financial viewpoint.

    » Project costs for new educational activities and initiatives.

    » Assess costs of current educational activities (Alspach, 1995).

PRIORITIZATION

▶ Be proactive rather than reactive in setting priorities.

▶ Base priorities on nursing service and organizational strategic priorities.

▶ Planning is key to setting priorities and managing time.

    » Determine goals and rank by time needed to complete planning and accomplish goals.

    » Identify plan; include human and financial resources needed to accomplish goals.

    » Work the plan.

▶ Organize activities to facilitate achievement of goal or outcome.

    Coordinate resources (people, equipment, and space).

    Provide authority and communication.

▶ Delegate, use deadlines, and create a sense of urgency.

▶ Follow up to ensure goal was met (Howard, 2009; Massello, 1998; Zimmermann, 2002).

▶ Alspach (1995) suggests basing priority on importance. To determine importance, consider:

    » High frequency (affects large number of staff)

    » High risk (harm to staff or patients if not done or not done correctly)

    » Problem-prone (produces problems for staff or patients)

RECORD MANAGEMENT

▶ See Chapter 12, Documentation and Records.

REFERENCES

Alspach, J. G. (1995). *The educational process in nursing staff development*. St. Louis, MO: Mosby.

American Nurses Association and National Nursing Staff Development Organization (2010). *Nursing professional development: Scope and standards of practice*. Silver Spring, MD: Nursesbooks.org.

Avillion, A., Brunt, B., & Ferrell, M. J. (2007). *Nursing professional development review and resource manual*. Silver Spring, MD: American Nurses Credentialing Center.

Blauth, C., & DeiTos, P. (2012). *Addendum to nursing professional development review and resource manual* (2nd ed.). Silver Spring, MD: American Nurses Credentialing Center.

Howard, K. P. (2009). Role of the manager in staff development. In S. L. Bruce (Ed.), *Core curriculum for staff development* (3rd ed., pp. 451–474). Pensacola, FL: National Nursing Staff Development Organization.

Massello, D. J. (1998) Operations management: Administering the program. In K. J. Kelly-Thomas, *Clinical and nursing staff development: Current competence, future focus* (2nd ed., pp. 337–364). Philadelphia: Lippincott.

Smith, D. S. (2002). Managing budgets. In P. G. Zimmermann, *Nursing management secrets* (pp. 42–48). Philadelphia: Hanley & Belfus.

Zimmerman, P. G. (2002). Time management. In P. G. Zimmermann, *Nursing management secrets* (pp. 20–24). Philadelphia: Hanley & Belfus.

CHAPTER 16

PROJECT MANAGEMENT

COMPONENTS OF PROJECT MANAGEMENT

▶ Nursing professional development specialists need to be well-versed in *project management*: the application of knowledge, skills, tools, and human resources to plan, control, and deliver a project on time.

　▷ The project manager role is to mentor and educate members throughout the process.

　▷ Project management requires the expertise of nursing professional development specialists to explain, educate, mentor, and provide additional perspectives of the project or process.

　▷ As the steps of the project are defined, nursing professional development specialists can educate members on what to expect, explain concepts, and create cooperative learning environments.

▶ Project management is different from program management.

　▷ Project management looks at the specific project from the beginning to the end.

　▷ Program management is usually longer in length and looks at multiple projects that are part of the program.

▶ Projects have three key objectives:

　▷ Meet the budget

　▷ Complete on schedule

　▷ Produce deliverables that meet the client needs (Mantel, Meredith, Shafer & Sutton, 2011, p. 8)

- ▶ A project can involve one person, a single department, or many or even all departments.

- ▶ A project can produce a:

  - » Product

  - » Capability to perform a service

  - » Result such as an outcome or document (Project Management Institute, 2008, p. 5)

- ▶ Recommendations for effective project management:

  - » Commitment by senior management to a project is essential.

  - » Strong project leadership must be present. The leader needs to be comfortable with both positive and negative feedback. Feedback needs to be communicated in a timely manner.

  - » Provide training. Basic project management training needs to be provided to both staff and managers. Short lectures and practice exercises can help involved parties comprehend the project management steps.

PROJECT MANAGEMENT TOOLS

- ▶ Outline the project specific process, start and end dates, and responsible party for each component.

- ▶ Gantt chart

  - » Graphical representation of the duration of tasks plotted by the progression of time

  - » Tasks or activities are listed on the left side of the chart and dates are listed across the top. Activity duration is then indicated with a horizontal bar according to dates.

  - » A useful tool for planning and scheduling projects

  - » Helpful when monitoring a project's progress

- ▶ Cause and effect (fishbone) diagram

  - » Graphical technique for grouping people's ideas about the causes of a problem.

  - » Illustrates the relationship between a given outcome and all the factors that influence the outcome (Arveson, 1996a).

▶ RACI diagram

  ▷ Describes the roles and responsibilities of various teams or individuals in delivering a project or operating a process.

  ▷ Processes or activities are listed down the first column. Roles are listed along the top row.

  ▷ The cells are completed for who is **R**esponsible, **A**ccountable or must **A**pprove (may also use Supportive), who must be **C**onsulted and **I**nformed.

  ▷ Especially useful in clarifying roles and responsibilities in cross-functional or departmental projects and processes (Value Based Management, 2010).

▶ PERT chart

  ▷ **P**rogram **E**valuation and **R**eview **T**echnique tool is used to identify tasks and time estimates of complex projects.

  ▷ Illustrates the activities that are performed sequentially and those performed in parallel

  ▷ Beneficial for determining time requirements of complex projects (NetMBA, 2010).

▶ Flowchart (flow diagram)

  ▷ Uses graphic symbols to depict the nature and order of steps in a process.

  ▷ Symbols used:

    ▷ Oval: Start and end points

    ▷ Box: Individual step or activity in the process

    ▷ Diamond: Decision point in the process (e.g., yes or no, go or no go); each decision has a path to follow from the diamond

    ▷ Circle: Step is connected to another part or page of the flow chart, indicated with a letter.

    ▷ Triangle: Place in the process where measurement occurs

  ▷ Benefits of flowcharts:

    ▷ Promote process understanding

    ▷ Provide tools for training

    ▷ Identify problem areas for improvement

    ▷ Depict process relationships (Arveson, 1996b).

IMPLEMENTATION STAGES OF PROJECT MANAGEMENT

- ► System selection of goal

    - ▷ Goal for the project needs to be specific to the project's overall focus

- ► Stakeholder support

    - ▷ Determine who the stakeholders are and consult with them often.

- ► Charter and scope of project team

    - ▷ Determine the scope of the project, funding source, and what must be achieved.

- ► Formulation of team

    - ▷ Identify team members who will ensure success as the project rolls out.

- ► Identification of risk

    - ▷ Identify strengths, weaknesses, opportunities, and threats (SWOT analysis) as the project moves forward. The goal is to minimize the risks.

- ► Requirements of the project

    - ▷ Detailed outline of the steps of the process

    - ▷ Include the start and end dates of each step

        - ▷ Follow up and provide constructive feedback if due dates are not met.

    - ▷ Determine the members' roles and responsibilities

- ► Training

    - ▷ Training for the specific project will be necessary. It is important to provide a variety of different training modalities for the learners.

    - ▷ Just-in-time training is training provided when and where it may be necessary. Examples:

        - ▷ e-learning

        - ▷ Education done at the time of the need

        - ▷ Review of a procedure or standard of practice regarding a situation of low incidence and high risk

- ► Evaluation

    - ▷ Goal is to have all the members be satisfied with the outcome.

    - ▷ Continuous evaluation should be done throughout the process. Evaluate progress at the end of each milestone or project process so adjustments can be made if necessary.

▶ Maintenance

▹ Change is perpetual. After the project is complete, the nursing professional development specialist may be responsible for ensuring continuous improvement to the system.

▹ System and staff are responsible for the sustainability of the project.

▹ Handoff strategies are critical because the staff assumes responsibility for sustaining the project

REFERENCES

Arveson, P. (1996a). *Module 5: Cause and effect diagram.* Retrieved from http://www.balancedscorecard.org/Portals/0/PDF/c-ediag.pdf

Arveson, P. (1996b). *Module 6: Flowchart.* Retrieved from http://www.balancedscorecard.org/Portals/0/PDF/flowchrt.pdf

Blauth, C., & DeiTos, P. (2012). *Addendum to nursing professional development review and resource manual* (2nd ed.). Silver Spring, MD: American Nurses Credentialing Center.

Mantel, S. J., Meredith, J. R., Shafer, S. M., & Sutton, M. M. (2011). *Project management practice.* Hoboken: John Wiley & Sons.

NetMBA (2010). *PERT.* Retrieved from http://www.netmba.com/operations/project/pert/

Project Management Institute. (2008). *A guide to the project management body of knowledge* (4th ed.). Newtown Square, PA: Author.

Value Based Management.net. (2010). *The RACI model.* Retrieved from http://www.valuebasedmanagement.net/methods_raci.html

CHAPTER 17

CONSULTATION PROCESS

BACKGROUND

▶ The nursing professional development "specialist provides consultation to influence plans, enhance the abilities of others, and effect change by:

  ▹ Synthesiz[ing] data and information, while incorporating conceptual or theoretical frameworks, when providing consultation

  ▹ Facilitat[ing] the effectiveness of a consultation by involving the learners, stakeholders, and members of other specialties in the decision-making process and negotiation of role responsibilities

  ▹ Communicat[ing] consultation recommendations that influence the identified plan, facilitate understanding by stakeholders, enhance the work of others, and effect change

  ▹ Establish[ing] formal and informal consultative relationships that may lead to professional development or mentorship opportunities

  ▹ Advis[ing] on the design, development, implementation, and evaluation of materials and teaching strategies appropriate to the situation and the learner's developmental level, learning needs, readiness, ability to learn, language preference, and culture

  ▹ Consider[ing] theories pertaining to learning behavioral change, motivation, epidemiology, and other related frameworks in consulting and collaborating when designing educational materials and programs

  ▹ Develop[ing] recommendations and strategies to address problems and complex issues." (American Nurses Association [ANA] & National Nursing Staff Development Organization [NNSDO], 2010, p. 30)

▶ *Consultation:* A process providing professional or expert advice or services

▶ *Internal consultant:* An employee within the organization who is in an advisory or support role

▶ *External consultant:* An expert brought into an organization to guide, educate, or coordinate the effort of an organization through a contractually negotiated partnership for a designated time (Jackson, 2002)

▶ ANA Standards of Professional Performance related to the consultant role

  » *Standard 5C—Collaboration:* "The nursing professional development specialist provides consultation to influence plans, enhance the abilities of others, and effect change" (ANA & NNSDO, 2010, p. 30).

  » *Standard 10—Collegiality:* "The nursing professional development specialist establishes collegial partnerships contributing to the professional development of peers, students, colleagues, and others" (ANA & NNSDO, 2010, p. 35)

CONSULTATIONS BY THE NURSING PROFESSIONAL DEVELOPMENT SPECIALIST

▶ Are dependent on experience and educational preparation

▶ Address various areas:

  » Care planning

  » Professional growth of others

  » Practice change based on evidence-based practice (EBP)

  » Clinical practice evaluation (ANA & NNSDO 2010, as cited in Hutchins, 2013)

Consultant Skills

▶ Expertise on the specific subject

▶ Communicate effectively, orally and in writing, to a variety of stakeholders

▶ Form consultative relationships

▶ Collaborate in decision-making

▶ Model critical thinking and problem-solving

▶ Synthesize and apply evidence-based practice and research findings

▶ Incorporate theoretical background to topic

▶ Formulate plans of action

▶ Implement educational program and clinical practice changes

▶ Build consensus

▶ Implement all phases of consultation process (Hutchins, 2013)

Contract Process

▶ A *contract* is an agreement that defines the purpose and goals of the relationship and delineates tasks, responsibilities, expectations, accountability, and the timeline for a project (Norwood, 1998).

▶ Components of a well-written contract:

  ▸ Statement of the problem and project goals

  ▸ Services to be provided by the consultant: tasks, methods, products

  ▸ Client responsibilities: tasks, supplies, resources, support they will provide

  ▸ Timeline with specific start and end dates; also may include interim progress reports or meeting dates

  ▸ Lines of authority, contact information, and communication expectations

  ▸ Confidentiality limits on consultant access to people and information

  ▸ Fees to be paid, expense reimbursement, and payment terms

  ▸ Process for modifying or terminating contract, including description of penalties

  ▸ Criteria and methods of evaluation and feedback

  ▸ Signatures and dates of acceptance (Jackson, 2002; Norwood, 1998)

Consultation Process

▶ Gain entry: Enviromental scan, contract, physical entry, psychological entry

▶ Identify problem

▶ Identify stakeholders

▶ Identify best practice, EBP question, or research hypothesis

▶ Develop educational program or EBP or research project

▶ Implement education program or EBP or research project

▶ Analyze effectiveness of process

▶ Identify additional related areas for consultation (Hutchins, 2013, p. 734)

Questions Before Starting a Consultation

▶ Questions for the consultant to ask the client:

  ▸ What results are you looking for?

  ▸ What do you see as the main problem and what has been done so far to address the situation?

  ▸ How long do you expect this will take?

  ▸ What do you expect me to do for you?

  ▸ What is the budget for the project?

  ▸ Who is involved in the decision-making and who are the key players? (Jackson, 2002)

▶ Questions for the client to consider:

  ▸ What do I want to happen as a result of the consultation?

  ▸ What am I willing to do to accomplish this?

  ▸ How much help do I want to accomplish this?

  ▸ How much time can I devote to the project and when?

  ▸ What resources can I provide?

▶ Questions for the consultant to consider:

  ▸ What do I want from the consultation—fees, other rewards?

  ▸ What am I willing to do to accomplish the goals of the consultation?

  ▸ How much time am I willing to devote to the project and when?

  ▸ What resources and support do I need from the client? (Norwood, 1998)

Preparing a Consultation Report

▶ Provide an overview of the problem: History, symptoms, challenges.

▶ Summarize the assessment process: Purpose, data-gathering methodology, sources, theoretical framework.

▶ Include data collected and tools used.

▶ Describe observations and findings as well as the process for analysis.

▶ Present conclusions and recommendations objectively.

▶ Provide an implementation plan and timetable.

▶ Summarize overall project process (Norwood, 1998; Puetz & Shinn, 1997).

Ethical and Legal Aspects of Consultation

▶ The ANA *Code of Ethics for Nurses* (ANA, 2008) provides a framework for ethical analysis and decision-making:

  » Practice within limits of licensure, certification, education, and experience.

  » Identify and avoid conflicts of interest.

  » Establish legal contractual agreements when appropriate.

  » Comply with organizational, state, and national regulations to protect patient safety and confidentiality (Hutchins, 2013).

  » Provide documentation of process and outcomes (Norwood, 1998; Puetz & Shinn, 1997).

REFERENCES

American Nurses Association. (2008). *Guide to the code of ethics for nurses: Interpretation and application.* Silver Spring, MD: Nursesbooks.org.

American Nurses Association and National Nursing Staff Development Organization (2010). *Nursing professional development: Scope and standards of practice.* Silver Spring, MD: Nursesbooks.org.

Hutchins, B. J. (2013). Elements of nursing professional development practice: Researcher/consultant. In S. L. Bruce (Ed.), *Core curriculum for nursing professional development* (4th ed., pp. 219–248). Chicago: Association for Nursing Professional Development.

Jackson, M. J. (2002). Consultant. In B. E. Puetz & J. W. Aucoin (Eds.), *Conversations in nursing professional development* (pp. 79–87). Pensacola, FL: Pohl Publishing.

Norwood, S. L. (1998). *Nurses as consultants: Essential concepts and processes.* Menlo Park, CA: Addison-Wesley.

Puetz, L., & Shinn, L. J. (1997). *The nurse consultant's handbook.* New York: Springer.

CHAPTER 18

FACILITATION

BACKGROUND

▶ The nursing professional development specialist acts as a facilitator by:

  ▷ Facilitating the learning process and actively involving the learner

  ▷ Assisting in the selection of teaching methods to accommodate learning styles and the learning environment

  ▷ Enlisting qualified instructors to plan, develop, and present (American Nurses Association [ANA] & National Nursing Staff Development Organization [NNSDO], 2010)

▶ The purpose of *facilitation* is to help people accomplish goals and keep systems running smoothly (Grasnick, 2002).

▶ The *Standards of Professional Performance for Nursing Professional Development* related to the facilitator role include:

  ▷ Standard 10—Collegiality: "The nursing professional development specialist establishes collegial partnerships contributing to the professional development of peers, students, colleagues and others" (ANA & NNSDO, 2010, p. 35).

  ▷ Standard 11—Collaboration: "The nursing professional development specialist collaborates with interprofessional teams, leaders, stakeholders, and others to facilitate nursing practice and positive outcomes for consumers" (ANA & NNSDO, 2010, p. 36).

FACILITATOR ROLES AND RESPONSIBILITIES

▶ Involvement with learning activities

 ▹ Encourage a positive attitude toward lifelong learning.

 ▹ Work with learners to identify learning needs.

 ▹ Plan activities to meet identified learning needs.

 ▹ Collaborate within and across the organization.

 ▹ Create an environment that is conducive to learning: comfortable, interactive, and distraction-free.

 ▹ Provide information and learning experiences using strategies that meet various learning needs and styles.

 ▹ Help learners to access internal and external resources, serving as liaison if needed.

 ▹ Provide feedback to learners (Brunt, 2007; Grasnick, 2002; Grey, 2002).

▶ Involvement with teams or projects

 ▹ Educate team members about team processes such as quality improvement methodology, tools and techniques, performance measurement, and data analysis.

 ▹ Help the team establish and maintain effective working relationships and processes.

 ▹ Work with the team to problem-solve, brainstorm, and contribute to the strategic learning process.

 ▹ Coach the team in methods of data collection, data analysis, problem identification, and the development of improvement strategies.

 ▹ Assist with the identification and involvement of champions and stakeholders who may influence or be influenced by the team and its goals.

 ▹ Help the team prepare for formal presentations.

 ▹ Work with the team to analyze the effectiveness of the team process.

 ▹ Provide support and encouragement.

 ▹ Use skills and knowledge of organizational processes to assist with removal of barriers or roadblocks (Brunt, 2007; Grasnick, 2002; Grey, 2002; Williams, 2013).

DEVELOPING FACILITATION SKILLS

▶ Observe facilitation skills used by others or create a mentoring relationship with someone whose facilitation skills you admire.

▶ Learn as much as possible about the work environment (e.g., ways to get work done, obtain supplies, or locate other resources).

▶ Learn how to use library, audiovisual, and Internet resources.

▶ Identify people who are willing to serve as resources when needed, including support staff and people from other departments with relevant skills and expertise.

▶ Check with people often to find out how they are doing and whether they need help or support.

▶ Set limits and be honest with others about what you can realistically do to meet their needs.

▶ Document the assistance that you provide.

▶ Seek opportunities to serve as facilitator to practice skills (Grasnick, 2002; Grey, 2002).

COMMON FACILITATION SITUATIONS

▶ Interdisciplinary teams

  » An *interdisciplinary* team is a group composed of individuals with diverse yet complementary skills and perspectives, formed to collaborate to achieve a common purpose or goal.

  » It may include representatives from clinical and nonclinical roles, leadership and staff positions, different disciplines, or other variations that bring individuals with the appropriate skills and knowledge to the group.

  » The facilitator ensures balanced contributions within the group and keeps the group productive and focused on the goals (Clark, 2003; Grasnick, 2002; Norwood, 2003).

▶ Focus groups

  » A *focus group* is 4 to 12 people convened to share opinions as part of an interactive, 60- to 90-minute discussion about a product, service, concept, or idea.

  » The facilitator's role is to lead the discussion by asking open-ended questions that encourage discussion related to specific objectives.

- The facilitator maintains the focus of the discussion, encourages balanced participation, and elicits honest opinions from the participants.

- An observer is present to take notes or record the discussion with permission of the participants (Clark, 2003; Cooper, 2002; Kitchie, 2008; Yoder Wise, 1996).

▶ Strategic planning

- The strategic planning process is applicable and shared at the unit, departmental, and institutional levels of an organization.

- The facilitator's role in the strategic planning process may include educating the team about tools and techniques as well as maintaining the focus of the group's work.

- See Chapter 2 for additional information about strategic planning.

▶ Meetings

- Meetings are used for participative problem-solving, decision-making, coordination, information-sharing, and morale-building (Tomey, 2009).

- Effective meetings have a defined purpose, are well-planned, and efficiently conducted to achieve the purpose.

- Preparing for the meeting

  ▷ Define the purpose and goals.

  ▷ Select participants, location, date, and time.

  ▷ Develop topics and time frames, and choose presenters or responsible persons and attendees.

  ▷ Distribute the agenda at least 24 hours in advance.

- During the meeting

  ▷ Start and end on time.

  ▷ Follow the agenda.

  ▷ Create a "parking lot" for side issues to be addressed later.

  ▷ Confirm action plan.

  ▷ Evaluate meeting effectiveness.

- After the meeting

  ▷ Recap decisions and assignments.

  ▷ Distribute minutes in a timely fashion (McNamara, n.d.; Tomey, 2009).

REFERENCES

American Nurses Association and National Nursing Staff Development Organization. (2010). *Nursing professional development: Scope and standards of practice.* Silver Spring, MD: Nursesbooks.org.

Apeles, N. C. (2009). Business and financial aspects of staff development. In S. Bruce (Ed.), *Core curriculum for staff development* (3rd ed.). Pensacola, FL: National Nursing Staff Development Organization.

Brunt, B. A. (2007). *Competencies for staff educators: Tools to evaluate and enhance nursing professional development.* Marblehead, MA: HCPro.

Clark, C. C. (2003). *Group leadership skills* (4th ed.). New York: Springer.

Cooper, D. C. (2002). Needs assessment. In K. L. O'Shea, *Staff development nursing secrets* (pp. 65–77). Philadelphia: Hanley & Belfus.

Cooper, D. C., & Bulmer, J. M. (2002). Staff development department management. In K. L. O'Shea, *Staff development nursing secrets* (pp. 47–57). Philadelphia: Hanley & Belfus.

Grasnick, L. L. (2002). Roles of the staff development educator. In K. L. O'Shea, *Staff development nursing secrets* (pp. 7–15). Philadelphia: Hanley & Belfus.

Grey, M. T. (2002). Change agent, facilitator, leader. In B. E. Puetz & J. W. Aucoin (Eds.), *Conversations in nursing professional development* (pp. 123–129). Pensacola, FL: Pohl Publishing.

Kitchie, S. (2008). Determinants of learning. In S. B. Bastable (Ed.), *Nurse as educator: Principles of teaching and learning for nursing practice* (3rd ed., pp. 93–145). Boston: Jones & Bartlett.

McNamara, C. (n.d.) *Guidelines to conducting effective meetings.* Retrieved from http://managementhelp. org/misc/meeting-management.htm

Norwood, S. L. (2003). *Nursing consultation: A framework for working with communities.* Upper Saddle River, NJ: Pearson Education.

Tomey, A. M. (2009). *Guide to nursing management and leadership* (8th ed.). St. Louis, MO: Elsevier.

Williams, K. S. (2013). Elements of nursing professional development practice: Educator/facilitator. In S. L. Bruce (Ed.), *Core curriculum for nursing professional development* (4th ed., pp. 339–357). Chicago: Association for Nursing Professional Development.

Yoder Wise, P. S. (1996). Learning needs assessment. In R. S. Abruzzese (Ed.), *Nursing staff development: Strategies for success* (2nd ed., pp. 188–207). St. Louis, MO: Mosby.

CHAPTER 19

CAREER DEVELOPMENT AND ROLE TRANSITION

BACKGROUND

▸ According to Standard 10 of the *Standards of Professional Performance for Nursing Professional Development*, "The nursing professional development specialist establishes collegial partnerships contributing to the professional development of peers, students, colleagues, and others" (American Nurses Association [ANA] & National Nursing Staff Development Organization [NNSDO], 2010, p. 35).

▸ The nursing professional development specialist may assist others in career development, role transition, and succession planning through counseling and providing activities that promote career development and role transition (ANA & NNSDO, 2010).

▸ The coaching process is an effective tool to help others reach their full potential as members of the team.

▸ *Coaching* involves a partnership through which one offers support, provides learning opportunities, nurtures others to build on strengths, and acts to help them succeed (Kelly-Thomas, 1998).

▶ The nursing professional development specialist may use coaching in the following situations:

⬧ Career development: Coaching to help people find jobs, advance in their current position, transition to a new field, or start a business

⬧ Clinical advancement: Coaching a learner in transition (e.g., student to RN, LPN to BSN, staff nurse to charge nurse) to encourage professional growth

⬧ Academic education: Coaching a learner to become socialized to the role of lifelong learner (Setter, 2013)

ATTRIBUTES AND ABILITIES OF AN EFFECTIVE COACH

▶ Maturity

▶ Self-confidence

▶ Enthusiasm

▶ Sense of humor

▶ Humility

▶ Optimism

▶ Assertiveness

▶ Empathy

▶ Trust and mutual respect

▶ Genuine interest and concern for others

▶ Tact

▶ Effective communication skills

▶ Open-mindedness

▶ Flexibility

▶ Goal orientation

▶ Resourcefulness

▶ Integrity (Ennis et al., 2005; Setter, 2013)

COACHING VS. MENTORING

▶ The terms "coaching" and "mentoring" are sometimes used interchangeably.

▶ *Mentoring* is a long-term partnership in which a more experienced person partners with a less experienced person to provide ongoing advice and counsel to guide career development (Zeus & Skiffington, 2002).

▶ *Coaching* is generally a short-term relationship involving an action plan to achieve specific goals for ongoing professional development.

▶ Some skills and traits are important to both coaching and mentoring relationships.

CORE PRINCIPLES OF COACHING

▶ Focus on improvement of job performance rather than changing personality.

▶ Use sensitivity and respect the dignity and worth of the person.

▶ Focus on the current level of performance.

▶ Provide feedback that meets the needs of the person being coached.

▶ Be specific and descriptive, not evaluative, when providing feedback.

▶ Coaching is most effective when it involves two-way communication and a free exchange of ideas (Marquis & Huston, 2012; Spangenberg, 2002).

Coaching for Career Development

▶ Combine coaching skills, role-modeling, and career management.

▶ Nurture new graduates.

▶ Discuss career goals and pathways.

▶ Give honest feedback.

▶ Identify developmental needs and resources to enhance current skills and learn new skills.

▶ Encourage, teach, sponsor, and guide nurses through significant career points.

▶ Act as a trusted, experienced counselor or guide.

▶ Celebrate successes (Avillion, 2004; Setter, 2013; Zeus & Skiffington, 2002).

Coaching for Clinical Advancement

▶ Discuss needs to transform values, beliefs, and behaviors from past experience to current environment.

▶ Establish goals to meet identified needs.

▶ Provide resources and opportunities for training.

▶ Encourage growth by reinforcing strengths and removing barriers.

▶ Celebrate successes.

▶ Encourage reflection.

Academic Education Coaching

▶ Create a culture that fosters continuing education.

▶ Provide information about academic possibilities.

▶ Facilitate study programs for groups of students.

▶ Inform current and potential students about available resources that support ongoing professional development (Setter, 2013).

ROLE TRANSITION

▶ Role transition occurs when a person leaves one role with a set of expected behaviors and enters another role with a different set of expected behaviors (e.g., student to RN, LPN to RN, RN to NP, staff nurse to nurse manager).

▶ The process of role transition includes several dimensions, including entry shock, role learning and unlearning, role innovation, experimentation, and developing and using social networks (Intergovernmental Studies Program, 2006).

▶ New graduate nurses experience reality shock in which they face conflict between ideals learned in nursing school and the realities of the clinical practice setting (Kramer, 1974, & Duchscher, 2009, as cited in Setter, 2013).

▶ Nurses transitioning into nurse practitioner roles experience extrinsic and intrinsic obstacles, turbulence, positive extrinsic and intrinsic forces, and role development (Heitz, Steiner, & Burman, 2004).

▶ The nursing professional development specialist assists nurses in role transition through orientation activities, nurse residency programs, and professional development or coaching opportunities that support the expected behaviors in the new role.

Succession Planning

▶ Succession planning is a process used to identify people for key positions within the organization (Setter, 2013).

▶ The nursing professional development specialist supports succession planning by:

  ▹ Identifying potential talent, considering clinical expertise, leadership, and individual success

  ▹ Facilitating professional development opportunities

  ▹ Designing comprehensive training and leadership classes

  ▹ Recommending mentors and coaches

  ▹ Creating role-related education

  ▹ Supporting practical experiences (Setter, 2013).

REFERENCES

American Nurses Association & National Nursing Staff Development Organization. (2010). *Nursing professional development: Scope and standards of practice*. Silver Spring, MD: Nursesbooks.org.

Avillion, A. E. (2004). *A practical guide to staff development: Tools and techniques for effective education*. Marblehead, MA: HCPro.

Ennis, S., Goodman, R., Hodgetts, W., Hunt, J., Mansfield, R., Otto, J., & Stern, L. (2005). *Core competencies of the executive coach*. Retrieved from http://www.theexecutivecoachingforum.com/docs/default-document-library/echb5thedition2_25.pdf?sfvrsn=0

Heitz, L. J., Steiner, S. H., & Burman, M. E. (2004). RN to FNP: A qualitative study of role transition. *Journal of Nursing Education, 43*(9), 416–420.

Intergovernmental Studies Program. (2006). *A practitioner guide to role transitions in organizations*. Albany, NY: Author.

Kelly-Thomas, K. J. (1998). *Clinical and nursing staff development: Current competence, future focus* (2nd ed.). Philadelphia: Lippincott.

Marquis, B. L., & Huston, C. J. (2012). *Leadership roles and management functions in nursing*. Philadelphia: Lippincott Williams & Wilkins.

Setter, R. (2013). Career development and role transition. In S. L. Bruce (Ed.), *Core curriculum for nursing professional development* (4th ed., pp. 515–525). Chicago: Association for Nursing Professional Development.

Spangenberg, S. L. (2002). When the problem is not an educational issue. In K. L. O'Shea (Ed.), *Staff development nursing secrets* (pp. 101–104). Philadelphia: Hanley & Belfus.

Zeus, P., & Skiffington, S. (2002). *The coaching at work toolkit: A complete guide to techniques and practices*. Sydney: McGraw Hill Australia.

CHAPTER 20

QUALITY IMPROVEMENT

PERFORMANCE MEASURES AND INDICATORS

▶ Purpose is to indicate

  ▹ Overall performance

  ▹ Progress toward achieving goals and objectives

  ▹ Patient and customer satisfaction

▶ Demonstrate process management

▶ Determine need for process change

  ▹ Review

  ▹ Reorganize

  ▹ Reinstitute

  ▹ Reevaluate

Core Measures

▶ In 1997, The Joint Commission released the ORYX initiative. It integrated outcome and performance measurement data into the accreditation process. Organization-specific performance data are used to guide the accreditation survey process and to monitor performance between surveys (Yoder-Wise, 2007, p. 202).

▶ Required by The Joint Commission for accredited hospitals

▶ Selection of data-driven measure sets from list of core and noncore measures

▶ Examples of core measures:

  ▹ Heart failure

  ▹ Acute myocardial infarction

  ▹ Children's asthma care

  ▹ Hospital-based inpatient psychiatric services

  ▹ Hospital outpatient department measures

  ▹ Immunizations

  ▹ Perinatal care

  ▹ Stroke

  ▹ Surgical care improvement project

  ▹ Venous thromboembolism

▶ Nurse-sensitive measures and indicators established in 2004 by The Joint Commission:

  ▹ Fifteen performance measures as managed by nurses

    ▹ Failure to rescue

    ▹ Pressure ulcer prevalence

    ▹ Patient falls

    ▹ Falls with injury

    ▹ Restraint prevalence

    ▹ Catheter-associated urinary tract infection (CAUTI)

    ▹ Central line–associated blood stream infections (CLABSI)

    ▹ Ventilator-associated pneumonia (VAP)

    ▹ Smoking cessation counseling for acute myocardial infarction

    ▹ Smoking cessation counseling for heart failure

    ▹ Smoking cessation for pneumonia

    ▹ Skill mix

    ▹ Nursing care hours per patient day (NHPPD)

    ▹ Practice environment work index

    ▹ Voluntary turnovers (added in 2005 by the Joint Commission; Fennel, 2009, p. 336)

▶ Patient satisfaction in today's competitive healthcare arena has elevated its importance as a quality measure.

▶ "The governance type is important to the nurse's work satisfaction and may be a determinant of the retention rate. Patient satisfaction is the consumer's evaluation of healthcare and service output and quality measures" (Strumpf, 2001, p. 196).

▶ "Correlations can be found in shared governance groups versus regular governance groups; conservative culture and job satisfaction, motivation, productivity and high-quality patient care" (Strumpf, 2001, p. 199).

▶ It can be concluded from the research study by Strumpf that patients report greater satisfaction with their care in shared governance organizations, which tend to have greater staff retention and work satisfaction.

   ▷ Care must be taken when focusing on patient satisfaction. Measurement flaws may exist that can skew outcomes:

      ▷ Designing a survey is difficult.

      ▷ Satisfaction is complex; expectations may not be realistic.

      ▷ Attitudes of patient and staff affect outcomes.

      ▷ Changes in levels of satisfaction occur over time, not immediately.

      ▷ Customers and patients must be considered as separate measurement groups.

   ▷ Patient satisfaction is currently focused on:

      ▷ The Patient Bill of Rights statements

      ▷ Knowing and understanding the diagnosis

      ▷ Knowing what treatment options are available

      ▷ Having appropriate care and services

      ▷ Pain management

      ▷ Improved progress

▶ Magnet facilities submit empirical outcomes data on patient satisfaction.

▶ The Joint Commission indicates the continuous quality improvement process activity of a healthcare organization includes outcomes of quality related to patient and customer satisfaction.

▶ Patient satisfaction data now have a prominent place on the unit and department report cards.

Report Cards

▶ Quality report cards are comparative summaries of health plans' actual performance against key indicators prepared at specific intervals and may be used to compare data from one organization to another similar organization, or to The Joint Commission core measures.

- Benchmarking may be an outcome of this process.

- Require careful interpretation

- Began with patient outcomes

- Developing further to include nursing

  ▷ Assessment of needs

  ▷ Skin integrity

  ▷ Patient education

  ▷ Discharge planning

  ▷ Patient safety response to planned and unplanned needs

  ▷ There may be additional information on patient days, RN education, RN certification, skill mix, and nurse turnover.

- More work on the value and content of a report card is required.

- Nurse knowledge must include comprehensive understanding of types of indicators and processes that offer the most distinct picture of patient and nurse outcomes.

Dashboards

▶ Dashboards, whether hard copy or electronic, offer a quick picture of data outcomes. Today and for the future, the world of electronics offers access to dashboards from many devices. Access to specific data pertaining to one or multiple dashboard topics is linked to a web page or application.

- Example: Patient satisfaction dashboard may include Press Ganey and Hospital Consumer Assessment of Health Plans Survey (HCAHPS) outcomes. A click on outpatient data or inpatient data links to specific and more comprehensive data outcomes for questions with patient responses.

  ▷ A Press Ganey Associates survey report of patient care delivery is used in many healthcare facilities to measure patient satisfaction, focusing on many areas of care delivery. The survey is sent to the home of the patient after discharge.

⊳ HCAHPS is a nationally standardized survey of patient satisfaction used to collect data on specific areas of patient care delivery that is prepared for public reporting. Generally a percentage of a facility's discharge population is sent the survey.

▹ A dashboard is the culmination of overall responses to a set of individualized questions that may include comparison to state or national outcomes or both, based on hospital size and available services.

▹ The dashboard is a quick reference to quality measures outcomes.

NURSE RETENTION

▶ Nurse retention by an organization helps it reach its mission and goals, especially quality goals.

▶ The purpose of recruitment is hiring staff necessary for the facility to provide safe, quality care.

▶ Retention is the strategy that allows the recruitment program to meet goals.

▶ Poor staff retention may indicate a need to reevaluate and revise recruitment activities to hire appropriate and sufficient staff.

▶ Recruitment requires thorough investigation of candidates:

⊳ Application review

⊳ Licensure

⊳ Background check

⊳ Certification

⊳ Prehire testing on campus

⊳ Behavioral interview

⊳ Interview with recruiter, manager, director (in some cases), staff on unit, and department

▶ Recruitment is costly.

⊳ Retention requires RNs and the environment to mesh cohesively

⊳ General and individualized departmental orientation

⊳ Culture and diversity of peers and patients

⊳ Addressing issues

⊳ Coaching

- ▷ Supportive administration

- ▷ Adequate staffing

- ▷ Autonomy and decision-making

- ▷ Innovative and invigorating environment

- ▷ Accountability

- ▷ Rewarding

- ▷ Recognition

- ▷ Respect

▶ Turnover issues annually cost organizations hundreds of thousands of dollars. Consider the cost of hire, orientation, salary, benefits, and advanced education activities. Also consider the effect on the remaining staff.

- Unit and department productivity changes

- Risks poor skill mix

- Increased frustration of staff

- Interrupted work team processes

- Increased responsibility of remaining staff until replacement hired

- Working with agency staff

- Potential instability of work schedule

- Preceptors and educators constantly orienting and educating new hires to unit and department

▶ How can managers and nursing professional development specialists help with recruitment and prevent staff turnover?

- Become actively involved in recruitment activities, on committees, attend career fairs.

- Provide a comprehensive orientation.

- Let staff know they are appreciated; support and encourage staff.

- Recognize contributions.

- Say "thank you."

- Build a wall of fame.

- Advertise certifications—a wall plaque in prominent view.

- Promote empowerment in self-scheduling.

- Assist with developing their career paths.

▹ Assess needs and follow up.

▹ Plan programs.

▹ Promote a safe work environment.

▹ Encourage, develop, and promote self-governance activities.

▹ Provide support, training, and opportunities for further education.

▹ Motivate those who are not self-starters.

▹ Create pride in the work of the unit team.

▹ Show respect.

▹ Be honest.

PROCESS IMPROVEMENT METHODOLOGIES

Six Sigma and LEAN

▶ Six Sigma and LEAN processes are quality improvement programs to evaluate measures to improve operational efficiency, which leads to cost savings. They often are used in combination to address administrative and service areas.

▶ Six Sigma

▹ Six Sigma is a process improvement method that focuses on eliminating defects by reducing variation.

▹ Six Sigma was developed in the mid-1980s by Motorola to determine strategies that reduced product defects. As short-term process improvements occur, the assumption is that long-term defect levels below 3.4 deficits per million opportunities (DPMO) will follow.

▹ Six Sigma is a statistical reference; it refers to the six standard deviations from normal. Six levels of sigma are defined by the DPMO and level of efficiency that can be achieved.

▹ One Sigma equals 690,000 DPMO or 31% efficiency.

▹ Two Sigma equals 308,000 DPMO or 69.2% efficiency.

▹ Three Sigma equals 66,800 DPMO or 93.32% efficiency.

▹ Four Sigma equals 6,210 DPMO or 99.379% efficiency.

▹ Five Sigma equals 230 DPMO or 99.97% efficiency.

▹ Six Sigma equals 3.4 DPMO or 99.99966% efficiency (Pocha, 2010).

- Six Sigma calculators are available for download or purchase to calculate the level of defect reduced. For example: If you have 5 medication errors per 100 medications administered, the sigma result is 3.5, or 50,000 deficits per 1 million. Achieving the desired outcome of Six Sigma would be equivalent to 1 medication error per 400,000 medication administrations, or 3 deficits per 1 million.

- Characteristics of Six Sigma

  - Systemwide data-driven approach

  - A business strategy

  - Concentration on those factors that are important to customers

  - A focus on eliminating defects or errors

  - Identification of sources of a variation and opportunities for standardization

  - Application of control to maintain the improvements

  - A structure methodology and approach to problem-solving

  - A powerful set of statistical tools (Lanhan & Maxon-Cooper, 2003)

- Members of the LEAN Six Sigma team

  - Master Belt levels

    - Black and Green Belt levels without a defined status

      - Black belts are usually the members who are responsible for the LEAN Six Sigma activity as a full-time position.

      - Green Belts are trained LEAN Six Sigma, but do not work full-time on the process.

    - Discuss the project with the leadership of the organization to determine the value of the project

    - Identify the appropriate person to lead the team.

  - Team sponsor

    - Member of the organization representing the leadership and administration

  - Team coach

    - Master of Six Sigma expert who will suggest the best type of tools needed for the process

- ▷ Team members

    - ▸ Persons who are involved with the process; all employees and customers should be included to create a multidisciplinary team.

- ▸ Deploys five phases that are followed in analyzing a problem. The phases are referred to as DMAIC (Define, Measure, Analyze, Improve, and Control).

    - ▷ **Define:** A problem statement is developed looking at supply, input, process, output, and customer (SIPOC), mapping the key quality characteristics of the problem.

    - ▷ **Measure:** Baseline data are collected throughout the process with validation of the system. Basic statistical data are calculated.

    - ▷ **Analyze:** Determine whether any disparity in the goal set and the current practice exists, using common statistical tools of graphical analysis, confidence interval, hypothesis testing, correlation, and regression and analysis of variation (ANOVA). Focus on understanding the relationship between cause and effect.

    - ▷ **Improve:** Solutions selected, evaluation of data, pilot trials, risk assessment, and implementation plans will lead to improved systems.

    - ▷ **Control:** The focus of this phase is to minimize variations in the process determined. Once the process is functioning to satisfaction, the ownership of the process is shifted to the process operators and teams.

- ▸ Tools and visual aids used

    - ▷ Pareto chart

    - ▷ Cause-and-effect diagram (e.g., fishbone)

    - ▷ Scatter plot

    - ▷ Histogram

- ▶ LEAN

    - ▸ LEAN thinking focuses on eliminating waste so all work adds value and serves customers' needs. Areas of impact include direct labor and productivity improvement, cost reduction, throughput and flow increase, improvement of quality (defects and scrap), inventory, space, and time. Focus on identification of bottlenecks in flow process and standardization of the work.

    - ▸ Associated with Toyota's production system and Japanese manufacturing.

- Requires the identification of value-added and non–value-added steps in every process, usually with a kaizen event: an intensive session focused solely on analyzing the current process and implementation of changes. Value-stream mapping of the process occurs during these sessions to allow critical evaluation of the process by all members.

- Requires commitment from executive level and all staff members involved to redesign processes to improve flow and reduce waste (supplies, time, or goodwill).

▶ LEAN Six Sigma in health care

- Utilized to help control healthcare costs caused by operational inefficiencies associated with the direct patient-care delivery process.

- Associated with the administrative, logistical, and operational side of the healthcare delivery system.

- Staff drives changes in the LEAN Six Sigma process.

- Effective LEAN Six Sigma creates stakeholder buy-in and willingness to

  ▷ Change daily practice.

  ▷ Adopt new and innovative ways to deliver patient care and alter aspects of the healthcare delivery system.

  ▷ Provide a method to systematically implement innovation projects in health care to improve performance and decrease the potential for errors.

- Overall, the system provides for methods of cost containment with input from all the key stakeholders or members of the team.

- The team rather than management decides what needs to be changed. LEAN processes promote shared governance in which staff decides what needs improvement, not management. This is a direct reflection of the principles of shared governance.

- Primary goal is to eliminate anything that does not meet customers' needs. To do so, one must know the following:

  ▷ What is critical to the quality of the product or process in terms of the customer?

  ▷ What is important to the customer?

> Nursing professional development (NPD) specialists' involvement is crucial to the LEAN process. They can:

> > Help to identify the bottleneck and work function correlation with standards of practice.

> > Assist with implementation in suggesting methodology on how to educate the change in new process.

Focus PDSA and PDCA

▶ Find a process to improve

▶ Organize a team

▶ Clarify current knowledge of the process

▶ Understand sources of process variation

▶ Select the process improvement

▶ Plan

▶ Do

▶ Study (or Check)

▶ Act (Gloe, 1998; Joint Commission Resources, 2004; Tomey, 2009)

IMPLICATIONS FOR NURSING PROFESSIONAL DEVELOPMENT

▶ "The nursing professional development specialist systematically enhances the quality and effectiveness of nursing professional development practice" (American Nurses Association [ANA] & National Nursing Staff Development Organization [NNSDO], 2010, p. 32). The nursing professional development specialist

> Is innovative in improving the learning experience

> Is guided by current evidence

> Effectively evaluates nursing professional development practice

▶ Performance indicators for nursing professional development are related to the orientation, inservice, and continuing education activities that assist nursing staff to develop, validate, and maintain the knowledge, attitude, and skills underlying nursing practice and quality patient care (Alspach, 1995).

▶ Outcome measures for nursing professional development are related to:

  ▹ Organizational mission, vision, and goals

  ▹ Initial and ongoing competency assessment

  ▹ Objective achievement and application to practice

  ▹ Adherence with educational standards (e.g., American Nurses Credentialing Center, The Joint Commission)

RISK MANAGEMENT

▶ Quality and risk management go hand in hand in organizations. *Quality* is determined by how well outcome standards are met. *Risk management* includes preventing and analyzing problems as well as minimizing loss after an adverse event occurs.

▶ Adverse events, never events, and sentinel events are reportable to The Joint Commission. Investigation of the events is essential.

  ▹ Identification and analysis of actual incidents and near-misses.

    ▷ Incident and occurrence reports are completed and maintained on paper or electronically, separate from the patient record.

    ▷ Near-misses are a sign of system issues or individual issues.

    ▷ Identification of near-misses helps the organization to correct system issues.

    ▷ Identification of individual issues helps to provide re-education for accuracy.

    ▷ Aggregation of incident reports assists in spotting trends in data to illuminate problem areas, improve quality of care, and decrease further risks.

    ▷ Incident reports should not be punitive in nature.

    ▷ The reports are not to be disclosed; hence, reference to their completion is not placed in the medical record.

  ▹ Adverse events are unintended injuries or side effects suffered by a patient, resulting in a medical intervention.

  ▹ A never event is a particularly shocking medical error that should never occur and is usually preventable. An example would be the wrong limb amputated in surgery.

▹ As described by The Joint Commission, a sentinel event is a serious, unexpected occurrence involving death or physical or psychological harm. Sentinel events are "special cause" variations, falling outside the normal central limits of the process of care. Intensive analysis is required when a sentinel event occurs in the organization or is associated with services provided by, or provided for, the organization.

> ▹ The Joint Commission has a sentinel event policy that sets a "community standard" for healthcare provider organizations:

>> ▹ Conduct immediate investigation

>> ▹ Report the sentinel event

>> ▹ Conduct root-cause analysis

>> ▹ Prepare an action plan

>> ▹ Present to The Joint Commission within 45 days

>> ▹ Implement improvements

>> ▹ Monitor outcomes

▶ The risk management department:

> ▹ Assists with defining the financial risk of errors

> ▹ Helps determine how frequently an event occurs over time

> ▹ Provides information when investigating events

> ▹ Provides information to plan appropriate intervention

> ▹ Recognizes the potential risks for events to occur

> ▹ Identifies opportunities for improvement

▶ The Joint Commission anticipates that healthcare organizations will educate employees, supply resources, and establish a program that will address potential failure mode and conduct an analysis annually. In conjunction with the nursing professional development educator, the risk manager educates nurses that every nurse is a risk manager in practice.

▶ A comprehensive risk management program includes

> ▹ Efforts to reduce events

> ▹ Reduction in negative outcomes

> ▹ Mechanisms to investigate events should they occur

▶ Risk to patient safety is reduced through use of one of several mechanisms:

  ▸ Failure Mode and Effect Analysis (FMEA): an evaluation process to determine risk potential

    ▷ Patient safety factors when planning a new process

    ▷ Patient safety factors in a current process

    ▷ Aspects of a process that could cause failure of the function or outcomes

    ▷ Required by The Joint Commission for certain high-risk incidents

▶ FMEA considers:

  ▸ Cause

  ▸ Effect

  ▸ Frequency

  ▸ Severity

  ▸ Probability

  ▸ Criticality

  ▸ Barriers to success

▶ The FMEA process, as led by risk management,

  ▸ Fully describes the purpose

  ▸ Establishes a multidisciplinary team (i.e., stakeholders)

  ▸ Educates the team on FMEA process

  ▸ Creates a step-by-step flowchart for activities

  ▸ Categorizes information

    ▷ The 5 Ps: people, provisions, policies, procedures, and place

    ▷ The 5 Ms: manpower, materials, machines, methods, and management

    ▷ Essential people, process, equipment, and environment (PPEE)

    ▷ Places information in a cause-and-effect diagram such as a fishbone

    ▷ Numbers to label each failure or potential failure

    ▷ Records courses on FMEA worksheet

- Ask questions, among them:
  - What is the outcome if any part of a current process fails?
  - What would be the outcome if any part of a process in planning fails?
  - How bad could it be? Rate it.
  - When could it happen (frequency)?
  - Where could it happen?
  - Why would it happen?
  - Who would be involved?
  - Redesign and implement to reduce risk
- ▶ Other risk-reducing mechanisms may include incident reports and events' root-cause analysis.
  - Root cause analysis (RCA) is a systematic process designed to
    - Dig down to the basic, underlying factors that contributed to the occurrence of an adverse or sentinel event.
    - Lend itself to a multidisciplinary in-depth analysis of all facets of the event and activities leading to the event (however, a multidisciplinary team is not required).
    - Address each level of causality, asking more questions.
    - Determine what, where, when, how, why, who.
    - Be a process of discovery that helps determine the impact on patients; patient care; location; players; process, whether system or individual; and other contributing factors.
    - Identify innovations for improvement: remediation via education, system process change, and policies and standards as parts of action planning.
    - Develop a monitoring plan: how, when, and what kind of data to be collected.
  - Incident reporting may be on hard copy or electronic safety reporting system.

REFERENCES

Alspach, J. G. (1995). *The educational process in nursing staff development*. St. Louis, MO: Mosby.

American Nurses Association and National Nursing Staff Development Organization (2010). *Nursing professional development: Scope and standards of practice*. Silver Spring, MD: Nursesbooks.org.

Fennel, V. (2009). Quality management in staff development. In S. L. Bruce (Ed.), *Core curriculum for staff development* (3rd ed., pp. 321–344). Pensacola, FL: National Nursing Staff Development Organization.

Gloe, D. (1998). Quality management: A staff development tradition. In K. J. Kelly-Thomas, *Clinical and nursing staff development: Current competence, future focus* (2nd ed., pp. 301–336). Philadelphia: Lippincott.

Joint Commission Resources. (2004). *Cost-effective performance improvement in hospitals*. Oakbrook Terrace, IL: Author.

Lanham, B., & Maxson-Cooper, P. (2003). Is Six Sigma the answer for nursing to reduce medical errors and enhance patient safety? *Nursing Economics, 21*(1), 39–41.

Pocha, C. (2010). Lean Six Sigma in health care and the challenge of implementation of Six Sigma methodologies at a Veterans Affairs medical center. *Quality Management in Health Care, 19*(4), 312–318.

Strumpf, V. (2001). A comparison of governance types and patient satisfaction outcomes. *Journal of Nursing Administration, 31*(4), 196–202.

Tomey, A. M. (2009). *Nursing management and leadership* (8th ed.). St. Louis, MO: Elsevier.

Yoder-Wise, P. (2007). *Leading and managing in nursing* (4th ed.). St. Louis, MO: Mosby

CHAPTER 21

RESEARCH PROCESS

BACKGROUND

▶ Standard 14 Research of the *Nursing Professional Development: Scope and Standards of Practice* states: "The nursing professional development specialist integrates research findings into practice" (American Nurses Association [ANA] & National Nursing Staff Development Organization [NNSDO], 2010, p. 40).

▶ Research competencies for the nursing professional development specialist identified by Brunt (2007):

  ▸ Supports integration of research into practice

  ▸ Incorporates research findings from a variety of disciplines into programs

  ▸ Accesses resources needed to facilitate research

  ▸ Develops and conducts research

IDENTIFY THE PROBLEM

▶ Cannot be general; must be narrowed to reflect a specific problem

▶ Guides the research process

▶ Must be clearly stated before research can begin

▶ Requires considerable thought, imagination, and creativity

▶ Must be significant, researchable, and feasible

▶ Needs to be an area of interest (Polit & Beck, 2014; Wood & Ross-Kerr, 2006)

Sources of Research Problems

▶ Experience: Immediate needs that are relevant and interesting

▶ Nursing literature: Regular reading of research literature can identify areas of interest, problems, or inconsistencies that need to be addressed

▶ Social issues: Global or local health care issues may suggest topics of interest

▶ Theory: Test applicability to nursing or nursing education

▶ Ideas from external sources: A direct suggestion from colleagues, faculty, employer, or funding agencies (Polit & Beck, 2014)

Searching the Literature

▶ Consult librarian for assistance if needed

▶ Access online databases for nursing, medical, and healthcare information (e.g., CINAHL, PubMed, Medscape, Nursing Center) as well as nonhealthcare resources if applicable to the topic area

▶ Helps researcher become familiar with current knowledge in area of interest

▶ Helps refine the research problem

▶ Determines if there are similar studies that could be replicated or refined

▶ May reveal previous methods that have proven useful in similar circumstances

▶ Can solidify need for or significance of research in problem area

▶ Use original (i.e., primary) sources rather than secondary sources.

▶ Needs to be comprehensive and include all relevant literature (Wood & Ross-Kerr, 2006)

Evaluating Research Articles

▶ Using the ASK (Applicability, Science, Knowledge) model

▶ Applicability

  ▹ Is this study relevant to practice?

  ▹ Do the findings suggest that the interventions tested made statistical or clinical improvements to practice?

  ▹ Does the benefit to the subject outweigh the risk of implementation?

  ▹ Is the change cost-effective in terms of human and material resources?

  ▹ Is the potential outcome for the subject or organization worth the effort to implement the change?

▶ Science

    ▹ The science is evaluated using standard criteria regardless of the practice area.

    ▹ "SPRMA" or "SPRTMA"—acronyms to help reviewers remember the key components of research

        ▷ **Statement** of the problem

        ▷ **Purpose**

        ▷ **Research** question

        ▷ **Theoretical** framework

        ▷ **Methodology**

        ▷ **Analysis**

▶ Knowledge

    ▹ Do the results fit the existing knowledge base?

    ▹ Do the research findings have meaning to the reader's knowledge base?

    ▹ Why wouldn't or shouldn't you use this idea? (Dittman, 2002)

Research Aims, Questions, Hypotheses, and Operational Definitions

▶ *Aim* outlines what the study is trying to achieve.

▶ A research *question* narrows the original problem to a more concise query that is measurable.

▶ *Hypothesis* is a statement about a relationship between two or more variables and predicts an expected outcome.

▶ The *independent variable* is the variable that the researcher chooses to control.

▶ The *dependent variable* is the outcome of interest or the variable that is affected by the independent variable.

▶ *Operational definitions* state the meanings of terms and how the terms will be measured (Polit & Beck, 2014).

RESEARCH DESIGN

▶ The research design guides the researcher in an organized fashion throughout the study.

▶ Strategies for sampling, data collection, and analysis of findings are determined by selection of a research design.

▶ A pilot study may be used to test the reliability and validity of data collection tools, or allow the researcher to practice research skills, such as interviewing techniques.

▶ Provides a plan or blueprint to answer the research question

▶ Internal and external validity are concepts basic to the issue of control.

  ▹ *Internal validity:* The extent to which the results of the study can actually be attributed to the action of the independent variable and not something else

  ▹ *External validity:* The degree to which the findings of the study are generalizable to the target population (Polit & Beck, 2014; Wood & Ross-Kerr, 2006)

Types of Research Designs

▶ Descriptive: Results in a description of the data, whether in words, pictures, charts, or tables, and whether the data analysis shows statistical or merely descriptive relationships

▶ Experimental: Results in inferences drawn from the data that explain the relationships between the variables

▶ Types of quantitative research designs

  ▹ *Experimental:* Subjects are randomly assigned to treatment or control group where the researcher manipulates the independent variable (the intervention, treatment, or condition introduced) and measures the effect achieved by the independent variable on the dependent variable.

  ▹ *Quasi-experimental:* Experimental treatment with a nonequivalent control group or no randomization, such as data collection before and after a treatment, or a time series design in which data are obtained from one group at several points before and after the treatment

  ▹ *Nonexperimental:* Researcher collects data without making changes or introducing an intervention.

    ▹ Exploratory: Provides in-depth exploration of a single process or variable

    ▹ Descriptive: Identifies characteristics of a specific population at one point

    ▹ Retrospective: *Ex post facto* studies in which the researcher identifies a current phenomenon and collects data from the past in an attempt to identify possible causal factors

▷ Prospective: Type of longitudinal study in which a group of subjects with a condition at present is followed over time to identify outcomes

▷ Correlational: Used to examine the type and degree of the relationship between two variables

▷ Case control studies: Descriptive study of a group of subjects with a condition compared to a group of subjects without the condition

▶ Surveys look at variables in a specific population or groups through self-report information.

▶ Needs assessments provide a basis for development of a policy or program.

▶ Methodology studies examine the validity and reliability of instruments (Hutchins, 2013).

DATA COLLECTION

Sampling Techniques

▶ *Probability sampling* uses random selection, with every member of the target population having an equal chance of being included in the sample; includes simple random sampling, stratified random sampling, and cluster sampling.

▷ *Simple random sampling* uses a table of random numbers to ensure that each unit in the population has an equal and independent chance of being selected.

▷ *Stratified random sampling* divides the population into strata based on the sample criteria, and then draws a predetermined number from each group using random sampling techniques.

▷ *Cluster sampling* involves repeated random sampling progressing from large to small units over two or more stages (e.g., choosing a selection of samples from home health agencies, then selecting a sample of nurse case managers in home health agencies).

▶ *Nonprobability (convenience) sampling* is selection without the use of random selection; includes convenience, quota, systematic, and network sampling.

▷ *Convenience sampling:* A minimum number of subjects or time frame is determined and everyone who meets the criteria is invited to participate.

▷ *Quota sampling:* Criteria to divide the sample into groups are identified, and then convenience sampling is used to fill the quota in each group.

   ▹ *Systematic sampling:* Selection of every nth number of the available population, after beginning with a random start.

   ▹ *Network sampling:* An individual or group meeting the sample criteria is identified, and the first and each subsequent member of the sample are asked to provide names of other individuals meeting the sample criteria (Wood & Ross-Kerr, 2006).

Data Collection Techniques

▶ Data collection methods are based on the hypothesis, research design, and characteristics of the population being studied.

▶ Methods of data collection

   ▹ Observation

   ▹ Questionnaires

   ▹ Interviews

   ▹ Available data

   ▹ Biophysiological measures

▶ Instruments must be reliable and valid.

   ▹ *Reliability* addresses consistency, stability, repeatability, dependability, predictability, and accuracy of the measurement.

   ▹ *Validity* is concerned with how well the instrument measures what it is intended to measure (Parker, 2009; Polit & Beck, 2014; Wood & Ross-Kerr, 2006).

DATA ANALYSIS

▶ Purpose of data analysis "is to reduce, organize, and give meaning to data" (Parker, 2009, p. 501)

▶ Types of data:

   ▹ Qualitative: Verbal, narrative pieces of information

   ▹ Quantitative: Numerical information

      Four levels of quantitative measurement:

         1. *Nominal:* Mutually exclusive variables are organized into categories that cannot be compared, such as gender or marital status.

         2. *Ordinal:* Categories are ranked by the interval between rankings and are not necessarily equal, such as levels of pain or educational levels.

      3. *Interval:* Equal numerical distances exist between variables, such as a 1–5 rating scale.

      4. *Ratio:* Highest measurement form expressing a continuum of values with an absolute zero, such as weight.

▶ Statistical analysis is used for quantitative data.

    ▹ *Descriptive statistics* describe data (e.g., frequency, mean, range, standard deviation, correlation).

    ▹ *Inferential statistics* draw conclusions about the population from relationships between variables (e.g., t test, analysis of variance, chi-square, regression).

       ▷ Existence: Does a relationship exist between variables?

       ▷ Magnitude: What is the strength of the relationship between variables?

       ▷ Nature: What type of relationship exists between variables?

▶ Data analysis can be about one (univariate), two (bivariate), or three or more (multivariate) variables.

▶ Data analysis is done for different purposes.

    ▹ Data cleaning: Done before analysis to find errors in data entry

    ▹ Sample description: Summarize sample attributes (i.e., demographics)

    ▹ Assessment of bias: Identify systematic biases (e.g., characteristics of volunteer subjects)

    ▹ Evaluation of measurement tools: Analysis of validity and reliability of instruments

    ▹ Evaluation of the need for transformations: How to handle missing values

    ▹ Addressing research questions

▶ When addressing research questions, statistical tests reject or accept the null (no difference) hypothesis.

▶ Type I error: Determine that a difference exists when in actuality no difference exists.

    ▹ Control for Type I error with "level of significance" (e.g., 0.05 or 0.01 levels of significance)

▶ Type II error: Determine that no difference exists when in actuality a difference does exist.

    ▹ Control for Type II error through power analysis (e.g., reaching sample size to a power of 0.80; typically determined prior to data collection)

▶ Biostatisticians can be helpful in determining sample size needed and identifying statistical tests to be done.

▶ Generally, a computer software program is used to analyze data.

▶ Create and follow a data analysis plan to decrease measurement error.

▶ Data analysis occurs during data collection to clean data, assess bias, evaluate measurement tools, and address missing data problems.

Interpreting the Results

▶ Explore significance of results.

▶ Describe limitations.

▶ Formulate conclusions.

▶ Identify implications and recommendations for future studies.

▶ Communicate findings.

  ▹ Descriptive statistics—narrative, graphs, tables

  ▹ Inferential statistics—narrative, tables

  ▹ Report to stakeholders

  ▹ Poster or paper presentations

  ▹ Manuscript (Parker, 2009; Polit, 1996)

INSTITUTIONAL REVIEW BOARD (IRB)

▶ Prior to implementation, all research should be approved by a qualified review board to ensure protection of subjects and ethical integrity.

▶ The IRB is a group that approves, monitors, and reviews biomedical and behavioral research involving human subjects.

▶ The IRB review process ensures that basic ethical principles are followed during the conduct of biomedical and behavioral research to protect the rights and welfare of humans participating as subjects (U.S. Department of Health and Human Services [HHS], n.d.-a). Issues of particular concern to the IRB are ethics, informed consent, confidentiality, and patient safety.

▶ Educational research typically falls under an expedited review.

▶ An expedited review can be done by the chair of the IRB or a designee rather than full IRB membership.

▶ Expedited review is used for research when:

  » The research poses minimal risk to the subject

  » Data collection is noninvasive

  » Data was or will be collected normally as a part of clinical practice
    (e.g., medical diagnosis)

  » Research is on individual or group characteristics or behavior
    (e.g., cognition, motivation, social behavior)

  » Research uses survey, interview, oral history, focus group, program
    evaluation, human factors evaluation, or quality assurance methodologies
    (HHS, 1998).

Elements of Informed Consent

▶ Purpose and procedures of the research

▶ Description of subject selection process

▶ Description of potential risks, discomfort, and benefits to the subject or others

▶ Statement of how confidentiality of records will be maintained

▶ Compensation, if any, is discussed

▶ Alternative procedures, if any, are disclosed

▶ Right to refuse to participate or withdraw from study without penalty is assured

▶ The IRB may waive some or all of the informed consent process when:

  » No more than minimal risk to subject is involved

  » Absence of informed consent does not adversely affect the subjects' rights and
    welfare

  » The research could not be carried out without the waiver, and

  » When possible, the subjects are provided with information after participation
    (HHS, n.d.-b)

REFERENCES

American Nurses Association and National Nursing Staff Development Organization. (2010). *Nursing professional development: Scope and standards of practice.* Silver Spring, MD: Nursesbooks.org.

Brunt, B. A. (2007). *Competencies for staff educators: Tools to evaluate and enhance nursing professional development.* Marblehead, MA: HCPro.

Dittman, P. W. (2002). Researcher. In B. E. Puetz & J. W. Aucoin (Eds.), *Conversations in nursing professional development* (pp. 89–101). Pensacola, FL: Pohl Publishing.

Hutchins, B. J. (2013). Elements of nursing professional development practice: Research/Consultant. In S. L. Bruce (Ed.), *Core curriculum for nursing professional development* (4th ed., pp. 719–748). Chicago: Association for Nursing Professional Development.

Parker, E. B. (2009). Researcher role of the nursing professional development educator. In S. L. Bruce (Ed.), *Core curriculum for staff development* (3rd ed., pp. 487–509). Pensacola, FL: National Nursing Staff Development Organization.

Polit, D. F. (1996). *Data analysis & statistics for nursing research.* Stamford, CT: Appleton & Lange.

Polit, D. F., & Beck, C. T. (2014). *Essentials of nursing research: Appraising evidence for nursing practice.* Philadelphia: Lippincott Williams & Wilkins.

U.S. Department of Health and Human Services. (n.d.-a). *45 CFR 46 - FAQs.* Retrieved from http://answers.hhs.gov/ohrp/categories/1562

U.S. Department of Health and Human Services. (n.d.b). *Informed consent – FAQs.* Retrieved from http://answers.hhs.gov/ohrp/categories/1566

U.S. Department of Health and Human Services. (1998). *Categories of research that may be reviewed by the Institutional Review Board (IRB) through an expedited review.* Retrieved from http://www.hhs.gov/ohrp/policy/expedited98.html

Wood, P. J., & Ross-Kerr, J. C. (2006). *Basic steps in planning nursing research: From question to proposal* (6th ed.). Sudbury, MA: Jones & Bartlett.

CHAPTER 22

EVIDENCE-BASED PRACTICE

BACKGROUND

▶ According to a measurement criterion in *Nursing Professional Development: Scope and Standards of Practice*, Standard 5, Implementation (American Nurses Association [ANA] & National Nursing Staff Development Organization [NNSDO], 2010), the nursing professional development specialist "uses evidence-based knowledge specific to the issue or trend to achieve the defined outcomes" (p. 27).

▶ In addition, Standard 14, Research, in *Nursing Professional Development: Scope and Standards of Practice* states that the nursing professional development specialist "uses the best available evidence to guide practice decisions" (p. 40).

▶ *Evidence-based practice* is practice in which clinical decisions are made based on the best available evidence, with an emphasis on research-based evidence (Polit & Beck, 2014).

▶ Evidence-based practice also has been described as a problem-solving approach that addresses a question by integrating:

　▹ A systematic search for and appraisal of the most relevant evidence

　▹ One's own clinical expertise

　▹ Patient preferences and values (Melnyk & Fineout-Overholt, 2010)

▶ Just as nurses are expected to use evidence-based practice in clinical practice, nursing professional development specialists need to base their practice on current evidence (Brunt, 2007).

> ▶ Nursing professional development specialists incorporate evidence-based practice through:

>> ▹ Integration of evidence-based practice into their practice

>> ▹ Facilitation of evidence-based practice as part of their role

>> ▹ Application of evidence-based practice within the educational process

DIFFERENCES IN EVIDENCE-BASED PRACTICE, PRACTICE-BASED EVIDENCE, RESEARCH, AND QUALITY IMPROVEMENT

▶ *Evidence-based practice* involves the use of the best, current, relevant, and credible research findings, clinician expertise, and patient preferences to make clinical decisions.

▶ *Practice-based evidence* involves the use of real-world clinical experiences to develop, refine, and implement high-quality, scientific evidence.

▶ *Research* focuses on generating new knowledge or nursing theory through the application of sound research methodologies to explore questions (Hutchins, 2013).

▶ *Quality improvement* refers to the ongoing measurement and evaluation of functions and processes to achieve quality care and customer satisfaction.

Steps of Evidence-Based Practice

▶ Step 1: Formulate the burning question in the PICO format: Patient population, Intervention of interest, Comparison intervention or status, and Outcome. May use PICOT format, including time frame.

▶ Step 2: Search for best evidence from a hierarchy of evidence.

▶ Step 3: Conduct a critical review of the evidence.

▶ Step 4: Implement the best decision by integrating the best evidence with the provider's expertise, assessment of the situation, available resources, and the patient's preferences and values.

▶ Step 5: Evaluate the effectiveness of the evidenced-based intervention in meeting the desired outcome.

▶ Step 6: Share outcomes of the evidence-based practice decision or change (Melnyk & Fineout-Overholt, 2011).

RATING SYSTEM FOR HIERARCHY OF EVIDENCE

▶ Level I: Evidence from a systematic review or meta-analysis of relevant randomized controlled trials or evidence-based guidelines based on such reviews

▶ Level II: Evidence from at least one well-designed randomized controlled trial

▶ Level III: Evidence obtained from well-designed controlled trials without randomization

▶ Level IV: Evidence from well-designed case-control and cohort studies

▶ Level V: Evidence from systematic reviews of descriptive and qualitative studies

▶ Level VI: Evidence from a single descriptive or qualitative study

▶ Level VII: Evidence from the opinion of authorities or expert committees (Melnyk & Fineout-Overholt, 2010; Polit & Beck, 2014)

▶ See Chapter 6, Issues and Trends, for additional information about evidence-based practice and sources of evidence.

ADVANTAGES TO EVIDENCE-BASED PRACTICE IN NURSING PROFESSIONAL DEVELOPMENT

▶ Provides high-quality, cost-effective educational services from a knowledge or evidence base

▶ Bridges the gap between theory and practice

▶ Supports the need for and stimulates interest in staff development research

▶ Improves staff development services to improve learners' job performance

▶ Enhances use of evidence in communication among departments

▶ Increases job satisfaction among nursing professional development specialists (Avillion, 2007)

Barriers to Evidence-Based Practice in Nursing Professional Development

▶ Shortage of research in the field of nursing professional development

▶ Lack of knowledge about the research process

▶ Lack of time for reading and evaluating research

▶ Lack of time for participating in the research process

▶ Staff resistance within the education department as well as by learners

▶ Cost to conduct research, analyze data, and implement practice changes (Avillion, 2007).

Integration of Evidence-Based Practice Into NPD Practice

▶ Create a positive climate for evidence-based practice and research in the practice setting.

▶ Disseminate current evidence-based findings through educational activities.

   ▸ Base educational programs and competencies on current evidence when possible.

   ▸ Discuss evidence and its applicability to practice in didactic or experiential learning activities.

   ▸ Conduct periodic reviews and update ongoing educational activities to incorporate current evidence.

   ▸ Include examples of evidence-based practice in the orientation process.

▶ Review course content annually to ensure it is current with the evidence.

▶ Maintain print or electronic files as you find evidence-based literature relevant to your work.

▶ Use current evidence in the development of practice documents such as policies, procedures, standards, and guidelines.

▶ Submit practice documents for periodic review to incorporate the latest evidence (Grasmick, 2002; Hutchins, 2013; Krugman, 2002).

Facilitation of Evidence-Based Practice as Part of the NPD Specialist Role

▶ Provide leadership in departmental activities that promote the use of evidence-based practice.

   ▸ Participate in research committees or councils.

   ▸ Collaborate with management, advanced practice nurses, and nursing staff to initiate and support evidence-based practice activities.

   ▸ Ensure that the facility's medical library subscribes to research and evidence-based resources relevant to nursing.

   ▸ Foster preceptor activities that promote valuing of evidence-based practice.

▶ Implement strategies that expose learners to sources of evidence.

   ▸ Post relevant evidence-based articles for staff to read.

   ▸ Establish a journal club for discussion of evidence-based articles.

   ▸ Invite colleagues to present evidence-based practice projects to staff.

▶ Mentor others in evidence-based practice.

▶ Offer a course on evidence-based practice (Melnyk & Fineoult-Overholt, 2010; Grasmick, 2002; Hutchins, 2013; Krugman, 2002).

Application of Evidence-Based Practice in the Educational Process

▶ Incorporate current evidence about educational process or strategies, educator expertise, and learner behaviors (e.g., teaching methodologies, learning outcomes, testing methods) into educational activities.

▶ Apply the steps of evidence-based practice to the educational environment.

  ▹ Question teaching strategies and educational practices.

  ▹ Search for best evidence.

  ▹ Critically review the evidence to determine whether it applies in this situation.

  ▹ Use the evidence to plan teaching strategies, evaluation methods, and other aspects of the educational process.

  ▹ Evaluate the effectiveness of methods (Melnyk & Fineoult-Overholt, 2010; Krugman, 2002).

REFERENCES

American Nurses Association & National Nursing Staff Development Organization. (2010). *Nursing professional development: Scope and standards of practice.* Silver Spring, MD: Nursesbooks.org.

Avillion, A. E. (2007). *Evidence-based staff development: Strategies to create, measure, and refine your program.* Marblehead, MA: HCPro.

Brunt, B. A. (2007). *Competencies for staff educators: Tools to evaluate and enhance nursing professional development.* Marblehead, MA: HCPro.

Grasmick, L. L. (2002). Roles of the staff development educator. In K. L. O'Shea (Ed.), *Staff development nursing secrets* (pp. 7–15). Philadelphia: Hanley & Belfus.

Hutchins, B. J. (2013). Elements of nursing professional development practice: Researcher/consultant. In S. L. Bruce (Ed.), *Core curriculum for nursing professional development* (4th ed., pp. 719–748). Chicago: Association for Nursing Professional Development.

Krugman, M. (2002). Evidence-based practice. In B. E. Puetz & J. W. Aucoin (Eds.), *Conversations in nursing professional development* (pp. 349–364). Pensacola, FL: Pohl Publishing.

Melnyk, B. M., & Fineout-Overholt, E. (2010). *Evidence-based practice in nursing and healthcare: A guide to best practice* (2nd ed.). Philadelphia: Lippincott Williams & Wilkins.

Polit, D. F., & Beck, C. T. (2014). *Essentials of nursing research: Appraising evidence for nursing practice* (8th ed.). Philadelphia: Lippincott Williams & Wilkins.

CHAPTER 23

INFORMATICS

INFORMATION MANAGEMENT

▶ Information can now be accessed at a rapid pace via the Internet and mobile devices thanks to rapid technological advances (Holtschneider, 2013).

▶ Mobile devices, social networking sites, blogs, and online learning tools provide immediate access to information and learning opportunities.

▶ Computer skills are essential for the nursing professional development specialist.

▶ The basic software programs on a personal computer may include word processing, spreadsheet, desktop publishing, graphics presentation, and business software.

▶ Word processing enables development of handouts, notes, and documents.

▶ Spreadsheets can be used to manage education budgets and maintain educational records.

▶ A desktop publishing program provides preformatted newsletters, brochures, letters, and labels, allowing for design of sophisticated fliers to market educational activities.

▶ Communication is enhanced by use of email programs, intranet, and Internet access.

▶ The Internet provides access to search engines (e.g., Bing, Google, Yahoo!) and databases for nursing, medical, and healthcare information (e.g., CINAHL, PubMed, Medscape, Nursing Center).

▶ Organization-specific information is exchanged through an intranet. Items on an intranet may include hospital newsletters, policies and procedures, laboratory manuals, and medical references. Employees are given access via user names and passwords.

▶ Other hospital systems also employ user names and passwords (e.g., medication and supply access, glucose monitoring devices, clinical information systems, email, access to medical references).

▶ One's role within the organization determines the level of access to these systems.

▶ The information technology (IT) department is the typical contact for assigning user names and passwords, as well as troubleshooting and resetting forgotten passwords.

▶ Learning content management systems are software for creating, managing, and reusing learning content (e.g., media, pages, tests, course components) as well as coordinating delivery and tracking of education (Horton & Horton, 2003).

▶ Nursing professional development specialists are change agents and facilitate staff acceptance of new technology (American Nurses Association & National Nursing Staff Development Organization, 2010)

INFORMATION PROCESSING

Collecting Data

▶ Data can be collected using paper, scannable forms, electronic health records, computer, a learning management system, or the web.

▶ Data can be collected from surveys, interviews, review of documentation, observation, focus groups, and case reviews (Warren, 2013).

▶ Data must be collated, organized, and presented in a fashion that allows interpretation and spotting trends.

▶ Data entry by hand requires time, cost, and "cleaning" for error identification.

▶ Scannable forms are paper-based but remove the data entry component. Design can include the familiar "bubble" and fill-in fields. Hardware and software are needed to read the forms and convert the data to electronic form.

▶ Computerized tests allow data to be scored, collated, and analyzed more readily than paper tests.

▶ Web-based surveys

　▸ Are less costly than paper surveys and questionnaires because reproduction, mailing, and data entry expenses are eliminated.

　▸ Data from web-based surveys are easily imported into spreadsheet or statistical software.

　▸ Requests and reminders for web-based surveys can be done using email with links to the survey embedded in the message.

Interpreting Data

▶ The nursing professional development specialist interprets data from tables, graphs, and charts, and applies that information to assess learning needs and evaluate outcomes.

▷ Bar graph: Displays differences of data characteristics; Y axis is frequency, X axis is attributes of the characteristic

▷ Histogram: Displays distribution of data; Y axis is frequency, X axis is range data, and bars are not separated as they are in a bar graph

▷ Pareto chart: Displays the relative importance of differences; the left Y axis is frequency, the right Y axis is cumulative percentage, and the X axis lists the attributes of the variable in descending frequency or magnitude

▷ Pie chart: Displays percentages of total for given characteristics

▷ Control chart: Displays process variation over time; Y axis is the variable scale, X axis is time

▷ Scatter diagram: Displays pairs of data to look for relationship (Polit & Beck, 2007).

▶ When looking at graphical or tabular data, read the labels or keys to assist with understanding.

▶ Consider equality of data and environmental circumstances at time of data collection when interpreting.

▶ Examples of data that the nursing professional development specialist interprets are patient, physician, and employee satisfaction; learner characteristics; quality improvement (e.g., handwashing compliance, core measures); course evaluations; and research literature.

Reporting Findings

▶ Data that the nursing professional development specialist reports include budget and educational activity information, test scores, course evaluations, performance reviews, and benefit–cost ratio.

▶ Qualitative data comes from interviews, focus groups, and open-ended questions on surveys and evaluations.

▶ The themes of qualitative data are determined from the data and can identify required action, provide descriptions, or support quantitative data.

▶ Qualitative data is typically reported in narrative form or descriptive tables.

▶ Quantitative data is numerical and can be reported in tables, charts, and graphs.

▶ Quantitative data for small groups is often aggregated.

▶ Reports are given to stakeholders and used for decision-making,

INFORMATION SYSTEMS

Clinical Information Systems

▶ Hospitals have a variety of information systems:

  » Electronic health record

  » Admission, discharge, and transfer system

  » Order entry, computerized physician order entry

  » Lab reports

  » Pharmacy medication dispensing robot

  » Automated drug dispensing system

  » Fetal monitoring system

  » Clinical decision support systems

  » Patient education software (Cooke, 2013)

▶ Clinical information systems may be fully integrated, partially integrated, or may not communicate between systems.

▶ Information can be mined from these systems to identify learning needs and evaluate learning outcomes.

▶ The nursing professional development specialist needs to identify what data are available and who can assist with access to the information systems.

Technologies for Learning

▶ Computer-based training: compact discs, digital video discs (DVDs), flash drives, Internet resources

▶ Content capture: videotaping and video systems that allow for marking key points and instant playback

▶ Conferencing technology

  » Teleconference using telephone to connect to different locations

  » Video conference with transmission of video and audio

  » Desktop video conference using personal computers

  » Web conference or webcast through the Internet

▶ Mobile device learning using smartphone, laptop, personal digital assistant, iPod, or electronic tablet (Hugget, 2010, as cited by Holtschneider, 2013)

- Electronic white board: participants in different locations simultaneously write and draw on an on-screen notepad viewed by others

- Podcasts (nonstreamed webcasts) viewed or listened to on computer or mobile device

- Learning content management system containing course content, tests, and evaluations

- Vendor-produced continuing education online courses

- Simulation including computerized patient manikin, computerized interactive programs, and virtual worlds

- Social networking sites including Facebook, Twitter, and LinkedIn create professional connections and have increased informal learning

- Audience response systems allow for participant input and participation (Holtschneider, 2013)

ENVIRONMENTAL SCANNING

- The nursing professional development specialist monitors progress, trends, and knowledge in areas of interest to her or his responsibilities.

- Outcomes related to education can be evaluated through quality improvement and risk management data (e.g., occurrence or incident reports, outcome data), course evaluations, medical record audits, feedback from managers, and staff attrition.

- Use technology to keep current with trends.

  - Websites
  - Electronic databases
    - Cumulative Index for Nursing and Allied Health Literature (CINAHL)
    - MEDLINE
  - Online Public Access Catalogs (OPAC; Holtschneider, 2013)
  - Medscape
  - Nursing Center
  - Specialty organizations
  - Listservs

- Specialty organizations and others offer literature scans in which you select topic areas of interest and receive emails with abstracts related to your topics.

▶ Newsletters from specialty organizations and nursing organizations provide timely content.

▶ Clinical applications are available on personal digital assistants (PDAs) and smart phones.

▶ Medical libraries provide access to current research.

REFERENCES

American Nurses Association and National Nursing Staff Development Organization (2010). *Nursing professional development: Scope and standards of practice.* Silver Spring, MD: Nursesbooks.org.

Cooke, M. (2013). Issues and trends in nursing professional development. In S. L. Bruce (Ed.), *Core curriculum for nursing professional development* (4th ed., pp. 587–613). Chicago: Association for Nursing Professional Development.

Holtschneider, M. E. (2013). Technology and nursing professional development. In S. L. Bruce (Ed.), *Core curriculum for nursing professional development* (4th ed., pp. 527–545). Chicago: Association for Nursing Professional Development.

Horton, W., & Horton, K. (2003). *E-learning tools and technologies.* Indianapolis: Wiley Publishing.

Polit, D. F., & Beck, C. T. (2007). *Nursing research: Generating and assessing evidence for nursing practice.* Philadelphia: Lippincott Williams & Wilkins.

Warren, J. I. (2013). Program evaluation and return on investment. In S. L. Bruce (Ed.), *Core curriculum for nursing professional development.* (4th ed., pp. 547–567). Chicago: Association for Nursing Professional Development.

CHAPTER 24

CONTRIBUTION TO THE NURSING PROFESSIONAL DEVELOPMENT SPECIALTY

BACKGROUND

▶ "The nursing professional development specialist evaluates his/her own practice in relation to professional practice standards and guidelines, and relevant statues, rules, and regulations" (American Nurses Association [ANA] & National Nursing Staff Development Organization [NNSDO, 2010, p. 34).

▶ "The nursing professional development specialist maintains current knowledge and competency in nursing and professional development practice" (ANA & NNSDO, 2010, p. 33).

▶ "The nursing professional development specialist establishes collegial partnerships contributing to the professional development of peers, students, colleagues, and others" (ANA & NNSDO, 2010, p. 35).

▶ The nursing professional development specialist contributes to the specialty by role-modeling behaviors that are hallmarks of a professional and engaging in professional interactions to support and advance the specialty practice.

ROLE-MODELING

Certification

▶ The nursing professional development (NPD) specialist "obtains or maintains professional certification" (ANA & NNSDO, 2010, p. 32).

▶ Certification of nursing professional development specialists provides recognition among peers and in the nursing community for attainment of a specialized body of knowledge (Lewis & Case, 2001).

▶ Additional reasons for NPD specialists to achieve specialty certification in nursing professional development include:

   ▹ Provides an opportunity to affirm knowledge and skills in education

   ▹ Serves as a benchmark for practice

   ▹ Demonstrates ability to function in a nursing professional development role, regardless of practice setting

   ▹ Creates a personal sense of satisfaction and goal attainment (Aucoin, 2002)

Competency

▶ The nursing professional development specialist "seeks experiences to develop, maintain, and improve competence in nursing professional development" (ANA & NNSDO, 2010, p. 33)

▶ *Educator competencies* are performance statements that originate from experience, observation, and validation and describe behaviors needed to fulfill NPD specialist activities and responsibilities (Wolff, 2002).

▶ Competencies identified by Brunt (2007):

   ▹ Designs and revises educational activities based on evaluative data

   ▹ Uses a variety of teaching strategies and material resources

   ▹ Uses and evaluates the effectiveness of material resources and facilities

   ▹ Conducts needs assessment using a variety of strategies

   ▹ Involves learners in needs assessment and outcomes identification

   ▹ Determines and revises priorities for educational activities

   ▹ Evaluates effectiveness and outcomes of educational endeavors

- Coordinates complex educational activities

- Selects appropriate teaching strategies to facilitate behavioral change

- Develops curricula using best available evidence

- Adjusts content and teaching strategy during presentation based on learners' reactions

- Creates and applies new educational methodologies

- Uses appropriate measurement methods to assess and document competence

- Possesses expert knowledge of how to teach within organizational culture

- Maintains responsibility for own professional development

- Communicates effectively with others, orally and in writing

- Develops and manages budget

Professional Self-Development

▶ The nursing professional development specialist participates in educational activities and acquires knowledge and skills as appropriate based on practice setting, role, and learner characteristics (ANA & NNSDO, 2010).

▶ Review job expectations and one's own knowledge base.

▶ Find a mentor, either within or outside the organization, to serve as a resource.

▶ Network with colleagues.

▶ Identify and act on one's own learning needs through ongoing academic or continuing education.

▶ Attend regional or national meetings in one's clinical or education specialty.

▶ Read journals and books in nursing, education, and related disciplines regularly.

▶ Set short-term and long-term goals and review on a regular basis.

▶ Participate in activities of professional and specialty organizations (Deck, 2002; Hood, 2002; Lewis & Case, 2001; Sturdivant, 2002).

PROFESSIONAL INTERACTIONS

Networking

- ▶ Networking with other professionals fosters professional growth.

- ▶ Establish networks with other educators within the organization and through involvement in professional organizations locally, regionally, and nationally.

- ▶ Electronic mailing forums (e.g., Listservs) provide a mechanism to establish a virtual network through which NPD specialists can generate discussion or share information about educational topics and trends.

- ▶ Networking provides a forum for the exchange of ideas and information to help the NPD specialist stay current about healthcare issues, clinical developments, educational strategies and trends, and political or regulatory issues that affect the practice of nursing professional development (Lewis & Case, 2001).

Mentoring

- ▶ The nursing professional development specialist "mentors colleagues, other nurses, students, and others as appropriate" (ANA & NNSDO, 2010, p. 42).

- ▶ Mentoring is a process through which a novice benefits from a relationship with an experienced professional who provides personal and career growth opportunities (Massachusetts Association of Registered Nurses, as cited in Harper & Rooney, 2013).

- ▶ A mentor can support, guide, direct, counsel, answer questions, provide feedback, and foster networking.

- ▶ Mentoring may be formal or informal.

- ▶ In addition to serving as mentors to staff nurses and others in the work setting, nursing professional development specialists may also provide educational preparation for mentors (Harper & Rooney, 2013).

- ▶ Novice nursing professional development specialists benefit from mentoring by experienced NPD specialists who can ease anxiety and facilitate integration to the NPD specialist role (Lewis & Case, 2001).

Dissemination

▶ The nursing professional development specialist "shares knowledge and skills with peers and colleagues through activities such as presentations at meetings and professional conferences and by participation in professional organizations" (ANA & NNSDO, 2010, p. 35).

▶ Publications

  ▷ Publication is one way to share innovative staff and patient teaching strategies that were successful in addressing educational needs.

  ▷ Writing for publication can be a source of personal satisfaction and professional advancement.

  ▷ When planning to prepare a manuscript for submission, read the journal's "Instructions for Authors" for guidance.

  ▷ Most editors of nursing journals are willing to work with authors to refine a manuscript into acceptable form.

  ▷ The *Journal for Nurses in Staff Development* (JNSD) and the *Journal of Continuing Education in Nursing* (JCEN), as well as other nursing and education journals, are publications to consider for submitting manuscripts about effective educational programs and innovations (Lewis & Case, 2001; Puetz, 2002).

▶ Presentations

  ▷ Presenting at meetings, conferences, and other professional gatherings is a way to share clinical and educational expertise and experiences with other nursing professional development specialists.

  ▷ Presentations may be formal (e.g., keynote speech, concurrent session) or informal (e.g., roundtable discussion, poster).

  ▷ The nature of a presentation depends on several variables:

    ▷ Your abilities and interests

    ▷ Needs and interests of the audience

    ▷ Your goals

    ▷ The nature of the setting (Paterson, 2002).

  ▷ See Chapter 9 for specific information about planning and delivering a presentation.

REFERENCES

Alspach, J. G. (1995). *The educational process in nursing staff development.* St. Louis, MO: Mosby.

American Nurses Association and National Nursing Staff Development Organization. (2010). *Nursing professional development: Scope and standards of practice.* Silver Spring, MD: Nursesbooks.org.

Aucoin, J. W. (2002). Preparing for certification. In B. E. Puetz & J. W. Aucoin (Eds.), *Conversations in nursing professional development* (pp. 375–378). Pensacola, FL: Pohl Publishing.

Brunt, B. A. (2002). Standards of practice. In B. E. Puetz & J. W. Aucoin (Eds.), *Conversations in nursing professional development* (pp. 365–372). Pensacola, FL: Pohl Publishing.

Brunt, B. A. (2007). *Competencies for staff educators: Tools to evaluate and enhance nursing professional development.* Marblehead, MA: HCPro.

Deck, M. L. (2002). Educator. In B. E. Puetz & J. W. Aucoin (Eds.), *Conversations in nursing professional development* (pp. 61–67). Pensacola, FL: Pohl Publishing.

Harper, M. G. & Rooney, E. (2013). Elements of nursing professional development practice: Educator/academic liaison. In S. L. Bruce (Ed.) *Core curriculum for nursing professional development* (4th ed., pp. 779–797. Chicago: Association for Nursing Professional Development.

Hood, A. W. (2002). Factors that affect the educator's role. In K. L. O'Shea (Ed.), *Staff development nursing secrets* (pp. 17–25). Philadelphia: Hanley & Belfus.

Lewis, D. J., & Case, B. (2001). The staff development specialist role. In *National Nursing Staff Development Organization, Getting started in clinical and nursing staff development* (2nd ed., pp. 92–98). Pensacola, FL: National Nursing Staff Development Organization.

Paterson, B. L. (2002). Presentation skills. In K. L. O'Shea (Ed.), *Staff development nursing secrets* (pp. 123–129). Philadelphia: Hanley & Belfus.

Puetz, B. E. (2002). Publishing. In B. E. Puetz & J. W. Aucoin (Eds.), *Conversations in nursing professional development* (pp. 391–397). Pensacola, FL: Pohl Publishing.

Sturdivant, M. (2002). Clinical. In B. E. Puetz & J. W. Aucoin (Eds.), *Conversations in nursing professional development* (pp. 103–111). Pensacola, FL: Pohl Publishing.

Wolff, A. C. (2002). Educator competencies. In K. L. O'Shea (Ed.), *Staff development nursing secrets* (pp. 27–37). Philadelphia: Hanley & Belfus.

APPENDIX A

REVIEW QUESTIONS

1. A staff nurse approaches the NPD specialist for advice about how to advance on the hospital's clinical ladder. Which aspect of systems theory in nursing professional development practice is represented by the NPD specialist's response?

    a. System feedback

    b. System input

    c. System output

    d. System throughput

2. Education about decision-making in a shared governance structure includes information about the:

    a. Clinical decision support program

    b. Human resource policies and procedures

    c. Organizational structure and resources

    d. Scope of shared governance council decisions

3. The ANA and NNSDO document *Nursing Professional Development: Scope and Standards of Practice*:

    a. Focuses on criteria that are useful in planning education that supports nurses in their professional development

    b. Establishes foundational competencies essential in the practice of nursing professional development

    c. Provides direction for the organizational structure of nursing professional development departments

    d. Reflects nurse practice acts, The Joint Commission standards, and federal regulatory requirements

4. Which situation represents a potential conflict of interest that must be declared at an educational activity?

    a. A conference planning committee member is an expert who has presented on the conference topic.

    b. A participant who works for Baxter mentions an infusion product during a small group discussion.

    c. A presenter discussing nursing care of cardiomyopathy patients is a member of Pfizer's speakers' bureau.

    d. At a class on ostomy care, the NPD specialist has a display table of wound care products in the hallway.

5. Which is the most important criterion for selecting an educational method?

    a. The method facilitates achievement of the learning objectives.

    b. The physical characteristics of the classroom accommodate the method.

    c. The teacher is skillful in, and comfortable with, the method.

    d. The time allocated for the learning exercise is sufficient.

6. Which of the following is the most appropriate annual goal for a nursing professional development department?

    a. All NPD specialists will participate in a quality improvement project to improve patient care in their clinical area.

    b. By the end of the fiscal year, 25% of registered nurses will complete requirements to become certified in their specialty.

    c. By the end of the year, a curriculum for a nurse residency program for novice medical-surgical nurses will be developed.

    d. The nursing professional development department will become more efficient and effective in delivering online education.

7. Which task is the responsibility of the mentor?

    a. Assessment of the work environment for the purpose of initiating change

    b. Development of a business relationship that does not involve socialization

    c. Establishment of a relationship between two equally qualified professionals

    d. Establishment of a relationship in order to provide advice and support

8. A preceptor complains that the preceptee is "just not getting it." After soliciting an example of the preceptee's behavior from the preceptor, the most appropriate action for the NPD specialist is to:

    a. Ask the preceptor to join the preceptor support group

    b. Discuss the teaching-learning process with the preceptor

    c. Interview the preceptee to gain her or his perspective

    d. Notify the nurse manager to take appropriate action

9. Which statement indicates an accurate assessment of a learning need?

    a. "Nurses on this unit state that they have never worked with unlicensed assistive personnel and need a class on delegation."

    b. "Our quality review data shows 10 medication events this month, indicating a need for a class on medication administration."

    c. "Tuberculosis cases in the state have increased, so we need a learning activity on tuberculosis transmission."

    d. "We have to teach the staff to use the patient care assignment sheets at the beginning of each shift."

10. Which action of the nursing professional development specialist reflects the use of best evidence from a hierarchy of evidence?

   a. Asks managers which topics they would like included in next year's competency assessment plan

   b. Includes results of a current evidence-based project on pain assessment and management in orientation handouts

   c. Revises course content annually when evidence-based practice guidelines have been updated

   d. Uses a pharmaceutical company's website to develop content for an educational activity on drug therapy

11. The nursing professional development specialist serves as a facilitator by:

   a. Creating a formal learning environment using information about learning styles to plan educational activities

   b. Directing team members to their manager if they encounter barriers to success in a care improvement project

   c. Having team members complete an evaluation tool to analyze the effectiveness of the team

   d. Volunteering to handle all data collection activities for a unit-based problem-solving group

12. One of the advantages of an institutionally based nursing professional development structure is:

   a. A central department facilitates coordination of education-related resources, programs, and support services

   b. An institutional department reports directly to administration, which facilitates decisions about educational priorities

   c. Centralized decision-making supports the allocation of resources to meet unit educational needs

   d. Institutionally based staff can more effectively meet the individualized learning needs of staff in multiple departments

13. Due to the nature of educational activities, the majority of research related to nursing professional development uses what type of research design?

   a. Correlational

   b. Exploratory nonexperimental

   c. Quasi-experimental

   d. Retrospective nonexperimental

14. The most comprehensive method for documenting professional competency is:

    a. 20 hours of continuing education per year

    b. Completion of annual competency checklists

    c. Completion of a professional portfolio

    d. Documented evidence of specialty certification

15. The nursing professional development specialist's area of responsibility includes 150 employees working on two patient care units. The most efficient and secure method for maintaining staff educational records is:

    a. A learning management system accessible to employee, manager, and educator

    b. A printout of an electronic spreadsheet posted in the locked staff workrooms

    c. Staff professional portfolios stored in each unit's staff conference room

    d. Unit-based files in the nurse manager's office on each patient-care unit

16. The nursing professional development specialist's cousin is a talented amateur photographer who has taken dramatic pictures of the buildings and grounds of the healthcare system where they both work. The NPD specialist is speaking at a national conference and decides to incorporate copies of these pictures in her slide presentation. What should the NPD specialist do to avoid copyright infringement?

    a. Access the photographs through the cousin's Facebook page to incorporate them in the slide presentation.

    b. Nothing, because the NPD specialist's cousin is not a professional photographer so copyright law does not apply.

    c. Obtain the cousin's permission to use the photographs before incorporating them into the slide presentation.

    d. Use the photographs in the slide presentation and tell the cousin about it when she sees him at a family event.

17. The NPD specialist is planning an educational event at which nursing staff will be recognized for their commitment to patient care and their safe patient handling efforts during the past year. This activity is most reflective of:

    a. ANCC CNE Provider status

    b. ANCC Nursing Skills Competency Program

    c. Healthy work environment

    d. Shared governance structure

18. Which of the following best describes a focus group convened to gather information?

    a. Eight staff RNs and LPNs meet for a 1-hour discussion with the NPD specialist about learning needs.

    b. Ten staff nurses are scheduled to attend a daylong conference to share upcoming changes in practice.

    c. The NPD specialist meets with a group of 12 staff members in various roles to administer a customer survey.

    d. Twenty nurses representing medical-surgical areas meet for 2 hours to explore the feasibility of a nurse residency.

19. The cardiology unit will be collecting patient data for a drug trial. To ensure integrity of the data, the nursing professional development specialist:

    a. Ensures the specific process for data collection is clearly delineated for staff

    b. Has the drug company investigator available for questions on data collection

    c. Has the unit's preceptors trained to oversee the data collection process

    d. Helps the primary investigator provide training sessions for the unit staff

20. The NPD specialist is working with a staff nurse to develop a plan for career advancement. This is an example of:

    a. Coaching

    b. Consultation

    c. Facilitation

    d. Teaching

21. The nursing professional development specialist applies the ethical principle of confidentiality through which action?

    a. Distributing a staff survey to gather needs assessment data

    b. Documenting the purpose and target audience for educational activities

    c. Recording the results of competency assessments on staff rosters

    d. Using a scanner to document attendance at educational activities

22. Return on investment (ROI) is defined as:

    a. An easy calculation process to determine the program value

    b. The process to determine degree of meeting stakeholder expectations

    c. The ratio of net benefits to costs

    d. The projected annual cost analysis

23. Which evaluation strategy assesses knowledge acquisition?

   a. A pretest and a posttest

   b. Calculation of program expenses compared to profit generated from providing a specific learning activity

   c. Questionnaire pertaining to the learners' perceptions of how well they were able to meet program objectives

   d. Skill return demonstration

24. The most appropriate sources for the NPD specialist to use for program outcome effectiveness include:

   a. Benchmarking and program evaluation data

   b. Dashboards and posttest scores

   c. Feedback from nurse managers

   d. Quality indicators from The Joint Commission

25. Resources for keeping up-to-date in NPD trends include:

   a. Apple Pages

   b. LinkedIn

   c. NPD textbooks

   d. Web-based electronic databases

26. An action that the NPD specialist takes during the "gaining entry" portion of the consultation process is:

   a. Completing an environmental scan to identify influencing factors

   b. Conducting a staff survey about barriers to attending educational activities

   c. Developing timelines and goals for achievement during the project

   d. Establishing an action plan for completion of the project

27. Generation X and Generation Y prefer learning activities that:

   a. Are classroom-based

   b. Are stimulating and interactive

   c. Integrate life experiences

   d. Take place in a formal learning environment

28. The NPD specialist determines the allocation of resources based on the:

    a. Expected profit margin

    b. Number of specialists in the department

    c. Priorities of nursing service and organizational strategic plans

    d. Projected length of stay of inpatients

29. A professional advantage for the use of social networking by NPD specialists is to:

    a. Discuss and debate issues related to education practice and research at a global level

    b. Teach staff nurses how to access social networking sites

    c. Improve computer literacy

    d. Integrate the networking site to a computer-based training program

30. The question "If you could transform your nursing unit in any way you wished, what three things would you do to heighten its function?" is an example of:

    a. Appreciative inquiry

    b. The first stage of problem definition

    c. Lewin's Change Theory

    d. The unfreezing phase of change management

31. The majority of management problems result from:

    a. Competing priorities

    b. Lack of communication

    c. Organizational complexity

    d. Time pressures

32. During negotiation, a win-win outcome is best obtained by:

    a. Bringing in a neutral party to mediate the issue

    b. Building understanding, support, and acceptance

    c. Compromising and looking for shared interests

    d. Empathetic listening and problem-solving

33. RNs and nursing assistants are in disagreement regarding roles and responsibilities for turning patients every 2 hours. A key component to assess is:

    a. How long the conflict has occurred

    b. The impact of perceived power

    c. The length of employment of each person

    d. The start of the shift

34. The process used to evaluate the potential risk of implementation of a new automatic medication dispensing system is a:

    a. Failure Mode and Effect Analysis (FMEA).

    b. Fishbone diagram

    c. Occurrence report review

    d. Strength, Weakness, Opportunity, Threat (SWOT)

35. The NPD specialist role is involved in risk management by:

    a. Counseling staff involved in events to encourage them to change clinical behaviors

    b. Determining the frequency and severity of events that have occurred in the institution

    c. Evaluating the financial impact of errors and potential cost-savings of error avoidance

    d. Planning educational content and activities that address gaps in practice and evidence-based practice

36. A recent handwashing campaign included posters, an online learning module with posttest, and huddle talking points. A nurse consistently enters a patient room without washing hands or using hand sanitizer. This describes:

    a. An educational issue

    b. A patient satisfaction problem

    c. A performance issue

    d. A process problem

37. The focus of the ANCC Magnet Recognition Program is:

    a. Empirical quality outcomes

    b. Improved hospital net revenue

    c. Physician satisfaction

    d. Senior nurse leader development

38. The education department is initiating a quality improvement project related to the inclusion of age-specific care concepts in educational activities. Which data source will provide the most useful data about this indicator?

    a. Chart audits

    b. Educational records

    c. Observation

    d. Test scores

39. Data sources for identifying learning needs and learning outcomes include:

    a. Admission, discharge, and transfer data and nurse manager interviews

    b. Course evaluation summaries and number of certified staff

    c. Clinical information systems and incident report trends

    d. Staff satisfaction scores and new grad retention data

40. To ensure current healthcare trends are included in educational activity content, the most appropriate action for the NPD specialist to take is:

    a. Conduct an annual review of the literature

    b. Review key websites (e.g., IHI, CMS,)

    c. Partner with the quality improvement department

    d. Have a colleague review the activity's slide content

41. What method is most effective for integrating congestive heart failure assessment, diagnosis, planning, and intervention that replicates a real patient case?

    a. High-fidelity simulation

    b. Podcast

    c. Web conference

    d. YouTube video

42. The IV Smart Pump data demonstrates 80% compliance for use of the drug library for the last 2 quarters. The goal is 90% compliance to minimize medication error risk. The strategy taken by the NPD specialist and nurse manger is to:

    a. Ask biomedical engineering to verify the accuracy of the pump data

    b. Continue monitoring the data

    c. Mandate all RNs attend 30-minute inservice

    d. Reactivate use of the Smart Pump use tip sheet

43. A tool that NPD specialists in different locations can simultaneously write and draw on an on-screen notepad viewed by others is:

    a. An electronic white board

    b. A learning management system

    c. A personal learning assistant

    d. A teleconference

44. The tool in project management that uses graphic symbols to depict the nature and flow of steps in a process is called:

    a. Flow chart
    b. Gantt chart
    c. PERT chart
    d. RACI diagram

45. The organization is changing to a new blood glucose meter. Key task force team members to ensure success are:

    a. Laboratory leaders, physicians, and financial officers
    b. Nursing directors and staff nurse representatives
    c. Representatives from laboratory, nursing, and pharmacy
    d. RNs representing different units across the care continuum

APPENDIX B

ANSWERS TO THE REVIEW QUESTIONS

1. **Correct Answer: D.** The NPD specialist is assisting the staff nurse to identify strategies to achieve her career goals, which is a type of throughput. The NPD specialist and the nurse (learner) are inputs. Outcomes of the learner's actions would be output.

2. **Correct Answer: D.** Information about the scope of the shared governance council's decisions is essential content for the group to learn about decision-making. Human resource policies and procedures and organizational structure information may be helpful adjuncts, but are not critical relevant to decision-making. Clinical decision support system information does not relate to shared governance.

3. **Correct Answer: B.** The ANA and NNSDO *Scope and Standards* is the foundational document that describes the practice of nursing professional development and delineates standards for this specialty area of practice.

4. **Correct Answer: C.** Commercial support guidelines identify that any faculty or presenters who have financial relationships with a commercial interest, such as being a member of a speakers' bureau for a pharmaceutical company, must disclose that financial relationship.

5. **Correct Answer: A.** Although the NPD specialist considers several criteria in selecting an educational method, the most important criterion is that the method is an effective approach to achieve the learning objectives. Classroom characteristics, time, and teacher skills can all be adapted as necessary.

6. **Correct Answer: C.** Development of a nurse residency program is an appropriate goal for a nursing professional development department. While NPD may be involved in quality improvement projects, they would be related to educational endeavors rather than direct clinical care. The NPD department has no control over whether staff achieve certification. Though increasing efficiency and effectiveness of online education is an appropriate goal, it is not clear how achievement of this goal would be assessed.

7. **Correct Answer: D.** The role of a mentor in a relationship with a novice is to guide, direct, counsel, answer questions, provide feedback, and foster networking. The relationship between mentor and mentee often includes a social relationship (option B). A mentor is a more experienced practitioner than the person he or she is mentoring (option C) and offers advice and support rather than directing change (option A).

8. **Correct Answer: C.** During the preceptor experience, the NPD specialist supports the preceptor by maintaining contact to guide the teaching-learning process, troubleshoot problems, and monitor the effectiveness and progress of the program. To do so, the NPD specialist needs to hear both the preceptor and the orientee perspective.

9. **Correct Answer: A.** Nursing staff members are an accurate source of needs assessment data when several staff identify the need and the need is validated by patterns of practice.

10. **Correct Answer: C.** Evidence-based guidelines are updated following a systematic review of current research and evidence on the topic, the highest level of evidence. Option A involves solicitation of personal opinion, the lowest level of evidence. Option B is action based on a single study (Level VI) and option D reflects use of potentially biased or incomplete information because the company wants to promote its products.

11. **Correct Answer: C.** The purpose of facilitation is to help others accomplish their goals and keep systems running smoothly. Having team members complete an evaluation tool is one strategy to assess system functions and improve effectiveness if indicated.

12. **Correct Answer: A.** A centralized department provides the opportunity for global coordination of resources and services. Not all centralized departments report directly to administration. Unit and individual learning needs are best met by a decentralized structure.

13. **Correct Answer: B.** In a nonexperimental design, the researcher collects data without introducing an intervention. Exploratory design provides in-depth exploration of a single process or variable. Professional development education typically does not allow the time or environment to introduce an intervention or multiple processes.

14. **Correct Answer: C.** The professional portfolio includes demonstration of learning and maintenance of professional competence. Continuing education, checklists, and specialty certification are components of a professional portfolio.

15. **Correct Answer: A.** Learning management systems automate record-keeping for job requirements, orientation, ongoing competency, and continuing education. Automation decreases time and error.

16. **Correct Answer: C.** The photographs are the intellectual property of the NPD specialist's cousin; therefore, the cousin's permission to use these photographs must be obtained. Other options given would be copyright infringement.

17. **Correct Answer: C.** A healthy work environment is one that is safe, empowering, and satisfying and a place where nurses feel empowered and valued for contributions to safe patient care. Options A and B are program activities of the American Nurses Credentialing Center.

18. **Correct Answer: A.** A focus group consists of 8–12 people who meet for 60–90 minutes to provide input about a specific topic or issue. A daylong conference and the use of a survey are not consistent with the design of a focus group.

19. **Correct Answer: A.** Clear, specific process steps for data collection enable consistent data collection. This is especially useful when a staff member misses training (option D) and when research investigators (option B) and other staff, such as preceptors (choice C), are not available.

20. **Correct Answer: A.** The NPD specialist uses coaching in several situations, including career development, clinical advancement, and academic education. Consulting, facilitation, and teaching are used in other aspects of the NPD specialist's role.

21. **Correct Answer: D.** The use of a scanner ensures confidentiality of participants' information. Option A involves documentation of aggregate data. Choices B and C are examples of documentation done within the educator's role.

22. **Correct Answer: C.** ROI is the ratio of net benefits to costs. ROI demonstrates the financial worth of a learning activity and is a complex process.

23. **Correct Answer: A.** Knowledge acquisition addresses the cognitive learning domain at the second level of evaluation. Tests are the most common measure of the cognitive domain.

24. **Correct Answer: A.** Tools to evaluate program outcome effectiveness reflect the congruence of goals, objectives, and accomplishments. Benchmarking compares accomplishments while program evaluations reflect goals and objectives.

25. **Correct Answer: D.** The most current resources for keeping up-to-date in NPD trends are web-based electronic databases. The other resources are less current or not specific to NPD information.

26. **Correct Answer: A.** Completion of an environmental scan is an important step in gaining entry before beginning work on the project or problem itself. The other steps follow later in the consultation process.

27. **Correct Answer: B.** Generation X and Generation Y prefer learning activities that are stimulating and interactive. Veterans prefer a formal learning environment and Baby Boomers prefer the incorporation of life experiences in learning.

28. **Correct Answer: C.** The NPD specialist determines the allocation of resources based on the priorities and plans of the nursing service and the organizational strategic plans. Priorities are reviewed annually.

29. **Correct Answer: A.** The professional advantage for the use of social networking by NPD specialists is to discuss and debate issues related to education practice and research with other NPD specialists around the world.

30. **Correct Answer: A.** The question "If you could transform your nursing unit in any way you wished" is an example of appreciative inquiry, which uses positive questions to seek possibilities for change and does not focus on problem definition.

31. **Correct Answer: B.** Communicating purpose, reasoning, expectations, and feedback are key to preventing management problems.

32. **Correct Answer: C.** A win-win outcome has both parties being comfortable with the result. Identifying shared interests guides negotiation toward those aspects each party can compromise on while maintaining mutual gains.

33. **Correct Answer: B.** A key component to assess when RNs and nursing assistants are in disagreement regarding roles and responsibilities is the impact of perceived power. According to PEPRS Framework, most participants believe that the other person or persons have the greater power in the situation. Other elements of PEPRS Framework are to assess persons, events and issues, regulation, and style.

34. **Correct Answer: A.** The mechanism used to evaluate the potential risk to patient safety when planning a new process is a Failure Mode and Effect Analysis (FMEA). A fishbone diagram and occurrence report review are done after a problem has occurred and SWOT is used as a process step in strategic planning or in project management.

35. **Correct Answer: D.** The NPD specialist role is involved in risk management by planning educational content and activities that address gaps in practice and evidence-based practice. The risk management department and nurse leaders have responsibility for the other options.

36. **Correct Answer: C.** The decision not to follow best clinical practices following educational activities is a performance issue. It is not a learning need or educational issue.

37. **Correct Answer: A.** The focus of the ANCC Magnet Recognition Program is empirical quality outcomes. The Magnet program recognizes healthcare organizations for promoting safe, positive work environments that promote the profession of nursing and quality patient outcomes.

38. **Correct Answer: B.** Educational records include information about themes and content of activities. Chart audits, observation, and test scores provide useful information for other potential quality improvement activities.

39. **Correct Answer: C.** Data from clinical practice records (clinical information systems and incident reports) provide objective information for learning needs assessment. Improvement in data from these sources will reflect the achievement of learning outcomes.

40. **Correct Answer: B.** Healthcare trends are reflected in industry initiatives. Websites of healthcare industries that affect practice are the primary source for current healthcare trends.

41. **Correct Answer: A.** High-fidelity simulation allows for the integration of complex skills, such as congestive heart failure assessment, diagnosis, planning, and intervention that replicates a real patient case. Debriefing as part of simulation is where the transfer of knowledge occurs. Web conferencing, podcast, and video are effective technologies for delivering information but do not include complex skill practice by participants.

42. **Correct Answer: D.** The data reflect significant compliance using the Smart Pump, demonstrating that the majority of RNs have the knowledge. Reactivating the tip sheet will remind staff of the expectations for 90% compliance and is a cost-effective approach. Ongoing monitoring has not affected compliance over the prior 6 months.

43. **Correct Answer: A.** The tool that NPD specialists in different locations can simultaneously write and draw on an on-screen notepad viewed by others is an electronic white board. Learning management systems provide opportunities to facilitate, coordinate, and track education. Teleconferencing allows three or more participants in different locations to discuss information using the telephone.

44. **Correct Answer: A.** The tool in project management that uses graphic symbols to depict the nature and flow of steps in a process is called a flow chart. A Gantt chart is a graphical representation of the duration of tasks against the progression of time. A PERT chart identifies tasks and time estimates of complex projects. A RACI diagram describes roles and responsibilities of teams or people in delivering a project.

45. **Correct Answer.** C. Key team members to ensure project success leading to change are representatives from the major departments affected by the project.

INDEX

INDEX

O

ABOUT THE AUTHORS

Ellen Gorbunoff, MSN, RN-BC, received her Associate Degree in Nursing from Pasadena City College, BSN from California State University – Long Beach, and MSN from California State University – Los Angeles, with a focus on nursing education. She has been certified in Nursing Professional Development by ANCC since 2010. Since 1996, she has served as the Director of Education and Professional Development at Providence Little Company of Mary Medical Center – Torrance. She has expertise in acute and post acute care nursing, interprofessional clinical and physician standards development, and education and nursing professional development. She has led the design, development, and philanthropic funding of two clinical simulation programs and oversees the RN Residency Program, clinical affiliation with nursing schools, and the management of numerous scholarship and nursing recognition programs. Ellen is the Chair of the Providence Health & Services Southern California, Education Optimization Domain of the Regional Nursing Institute.

She is an Assistant Clinical Professor, UCLA School of Nursing, and precepts MSN students. Ellen was Chair of the Nursing Leadership Development Committee for the Association of California Nurse Leaders (ACNL) for 2011–2012 and is a current member of the Association for Nursing Professional Development, ACNL, American Society of Pain Management Nurses, and Sigma Theta Tau.

Patricia Kummeth, MSN, RN-BC, received her baccalaureate degree from the College of Saint Teresa, Winona, Minnesota, and her master's degree in Adult Health Nursing with a focus in education from the University of Wisconsin – Eau Claire. Much of her nursing career has been spent as a Nursing Education Specialist in the Department of Nursing, Mayo Clinic, Rochester, Minnesota. In that role, she has been responsible for all aspects of the educational process from planning through evaluation of orientation, inservice, and continuing education activities for nurses. Now semi-retired, Patti has continued her involvement in nursing education as a supplemental Nursing Education Specialist at Mayo and teaching education-related courses at Winona State University.

In addition, Patti has served as a nurse planner for both Mayo Continuing Nursing Education and the Minnesota Nurses Association ANCC Provider Units. She has been an accreditation appraiser for the American Nurses Credentialing Center Accreditation Program since 1999. She was a member of the ANCC Commission on Accreditation from 1999 to 2002 and the Accreditation Review Committee from 2003 to 2010. She has been certified in Nursing Professional Development through the American Nurses Credentialing Center since 1992 and is currently an ANCC study group presenter for the NPD exam.

Made in the USA
Charleston, SC
11 February 2015